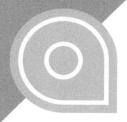

MYplace

FOR BIBLE STUDY

Published by First Place for Health
Galveston, Texas, USA
www.firstplaceforhealth.com
Printed in the USA

ISBN: 978-1-942425-51-9

CONTENTS

MY PLACE FOR BIBLE STUDY
Training for Success

FOREWORD

I was introduced to First Place for Health in 1993 by my mother-in-law, who had great concern for the welfare of her grandchildren. I was overweight and overwrought! God used that first Bible study to start me on my journey to health, wellness, and a life of balance.

Our desire at First Place for Health is for you to begin that same journey. We want you to experience the freedom that comes from an intimate relationship with Jesus Christ and witness His love for you through reading your Bible and through prayer. To this end, we have designed each day's study (which will take about fifteen to twenty minutes to complete) to help you discover the deep truths of the Bible. Also included is a weekly Bible memory verse to help you hide God's Word in your heart. As you start focusing on these truths, God will begin a great work in you.

At the beginning of Jesus' ministry, when He was teaching from the book of Isaiah, He said to the people, "The Spirit of the Lord is on me, because he has anointed me to preach good news to the poor. He has sent me to proclaim freedom for the prisoners and recovery of sight for the blind, to release the oppressed, to proclaim the year of the Lord's favor" (Luke 4:18–19). Jesus came to set us free—whether that is from the chains of compulsivity, addiction, gluttony, overeating, under eating, or just plain unbelief. It is our prayer that He will bring freedom to your heart so you may experience abundant life.

God bless you as you begin this journey toward a life of liberty.

Vicki Heath, First Place for Health National Director

ABOUT THE AUTHOR

Janet Holm McHenry is a national speaker and award-winning author of 25 books—seven related to prayer, including *PrayerWalk, PrayerStreaming*, and *The Complete Guide to the Prayers of Jesus*. Her prayerwalking practices have been featured in national magazines such as *Health, Woman's Day, Catholic Digest, Today's Christian Woman*, and *First*, and she has been interviewed widely on national and local radio programs about prayer. Janet has enjoyed speaking at conferences around the country. She has organized a county-wide prayer conference, has served as county chair for Moms in Touch International, has organized and spoken at Bible Girls conferences, organizes an annual prayerwalk for the schools in Reno, and founded and directs the prayer ministry at The Bridge Church in Reno, where she has been a First Place for Health member for more than ten years. In fact, her story was featured on the First Place for Health website, and she speaks often at First Place events. A high school English teacher and academic advisor, she and her husband, Craig, have raised four adult children in the Sierra Valley in northeast California. There Janet continues to prayerwalk on behalf of her community. She offers a free e-book called *Prayer Helps: Scripture-Based Prayers When You Don't Know How to Pray* on her website: janetmchenry.com.

ABOUT THE CONTRIBUTOR

Lisa Lewis, who provided the menus and recipes in this study, is the author of *Healthy Happy Cooking*. Lisa's cooking skills have been a part of First Place for Health wellness weeks and other events for many years. She provided recipes for fifteen of the First Place for Health Bible studies and is a contributing author in *Better Together* and *Healthy Holiday Living*. She partners with community networks, including the Real Food Project, to bring healthy cooking classes to underserved areas. She is dedicated to bringing people together around the dinner table with healthy, delicious meals that are easy to prepare. Lisa lives in Galveston and is married to John. They have three children: Tal, Hunter, and Harper. Visit www.healthyhappycook.com for more delicious inspiration.

INTRODUCTION

First Place for Health is a Christ-centered health program that emphasizes balance in the physical, mental, emotional, and spiritual areas of life. The First Place for Health program is meant to be a daily process. As we learn to keep Christ first in our lives, we will find that He is the One who satisfies our hunger and our every need.

This Bible study is designed to be used in conjunction with the First Place for Health program but can be beneficial for anyone interested in obtaining a balanced lifestyle. The Bible study has been created in a seven-day format, with the last two days reserved for reflection on the material studied. Keep in mind that the ultimate goal of studying the Bible is not only for knowledge but also for application and a changed life. Don't feel anxious if you can't seem to find the correct answer. Many times, the Word will speak differently to different people, depending on where they are in their walk with God and the season of life they are experiencing. Be prepared to discuss with your fellow First Place for Health members what you learned that week through your study.

There are some additional components included with this study that will be helpful as you pursue the goal of giving Christ first place in every area of your life:

o **Leader Discussion Guide:** This discussion guide is provided to help the First Place for Health leader guide a group through this Bible study. It includes ideas for facilitating a First Place for Health class discussion for each week of the Bible study.

o **Jump Start Recipes:** There are seven days of recipes--breakfast, lunch and dinner-- to get you started.

o **Steps for Spiritual Growth:** This section will provide you with some basic tips for how to memorize Scripture and make it a part of your life, establish a quiet time with God each day, and share your faith with others..

o **First Place for Health Member Survey:** Fill this out and bring it to your first meeting. This information will help your leader know your interests and talents.

o **Personal Weight and Measurement Record:** Use this form to keep a record of your weight loss. Record any loss or gain on the chart after the weigh-in at each week's meeting.

o **Weekly Prayer Partner Forms:** Fill out this form before class and place it into a basket during the class meeting. After class, you will draw out a prayer request form, and this will be your prayer partner for the week. Try to call or email the person sometime before the next class meeting to encourage that person.

o **100-Mile Club:** A worthy goal we encourage is for you to complete 100 miles of exercise during your time in First Place for Health. There are many activities listed on the 100-mile club pages at the back of this book that count toward your goal of 100 miles and a handy tracker to track your miles.

o **Live It Trackers:** Your Live It Tracker is to be completed at home and turned in to your leader at your weekly First Place for Health meeting. The Tracker is designed to help you practice mindfulness and stay accountable with regard to your eating and exercise habits.

WEEK ONE: TRAINING IN DEVOTION

SCRIPTURE MEMORY VERSE
Very early in the morning, while it was still dark, Jesus got up, left the house and went off to a solitary place, where he prayed. Mark 1:35

Do you want to make lasting changes in your life? Changes that others will notice and that will change you from the inside out? All of us want to be stronger and more physically fit, but if we have any experience with diet and health programs, we know changes that stick over the months and years have to begin with character transformation.

Sometimes, another person can inspire us to better ourselves. For example, we might have the benefit of a personal trainer to coach us in our diet and exercise routines. A personal trainer can challenge us to work out harder so we become more faithful and disciplined in our daily practices. However, not all of us can afford to hire a personal trainer, especially if we seem to need one 24/7!

The best person who could coach us—the one we will call our Personal Trainer in this study—is Jesus Christ. While He was fully God, He was also fully man during his thirty-some years on this earth. In fact, Jesus faced the same kinds of temptations, disappointments, struggles, and hurts that we do today. Yet in spite of the challenges He faced, His life was purposeful and victorious—and His personal traits, as conveyed through His life and teachings, still inspire us today. The best thing about having Christ as a Personal Trainer is that he is available 24/7—through the Bible and prayer.

During the next ten weeks we will examine a different characteristic we see demonstrated in Jesus Christ. This week, we will study His devotion—especially as it applies to prayer and memorizing Scripture. Just as Christ's devotional practices carried Him through the challenges of His days, the same kinds of disciplines can make us fitter spiritually, mentally, emotionally, and physically.

—— DAY 1: PRAY CONTINUALLY

Lord Jesus, Your life is an inspiration to me as I seek change in my life. Help me to become a more devoted person as I learn more about You this week. In Your name, amen.

To what are you devoted? *Devotion* is a sincere attachment or dedication to a cause, an individual, or a personal practice. If we seek to lead healthier lives, we will want to become more devoted to healthy eating and regular exercise—but we will also want to finish this lifelong race as more devoted followers of Christ. Prayer is an important practice in this, because it allows us to enter into conversation with our heavenly Father. Through a daily practice of prayer, we become more connected to and devoted to God. Read Mark 1:21-35. What tasks did Jesus do the day before going "off to a solitary place" (v. 35) to pray?

_____

_____

_____

Why do you think Jesus got up early that day and went off by Himself to pray?

_____

_____

_____

Read Mark 1:36-39. What pressures did Christ face in seeking a quiet place to pray (see v. 37)?

_____

_____

_____

Think about your personal practice of prayer. When and where do you pray? Under what circumstances do you pray?

_____

_____

_____

Although Christ prayed in the early morning in this passage, other verses show He also prayed at night and at different times (see Matthew 14:23; Luke 6:12). Whatever consistent practice works for you is the right one for you. Do you need a more regular prayer time? If so, describe when and where you could devote more time to prayer.

What kinds of schedule changes or commitments will you need to make so this prayer time works for you on a daily basis?

_____

_____

_____

What prayer requests relate to your First Place for Health journey?

_____

_____

_____

Dear Father, I am thankful that I can take my concerns to You at any time. Help me to develop spiritual disciplines in my life that will make me a more devoted person. In Jesus's name, amen.

—— DAY 2: PRAY SIMPLY

Lord, it is often hard for me to express to You the feelings and needs I have. Help me to remember that I don't need elaborate prayers for You to hear me. In Jesus's name, amen.

Sometimes we might think that because we are communicating with the most high God, we need to make long speeches in flowery language. Actually, the opposite is true. In Jesus's day the word *pagan* was used to describe people who did not follow either Judaism or Christianity. Pagans were people who either were non-religious, followed idols, or worshiped things such as the sun. Read Matthew 6:7-13. How did Jesus say pagans pray (see verse 7)?

_____

_____

_____

Why did Jesus say not to pray as they do (see verse 8)?

_____

_____

_____

Jesus followed this instruction with an example of a simple prayer—one that we now call the Lord's Prayer (see verses 9-13). Jesus began by addressing His Father in heaven and then offered a simple statement of adoration: "Hallowed be your name." In this way Jesus demonstrated we should start our prayers with praise and an acknowledgement that our Lord is the God in heaven. What requests does Jesus then make (see verses 11-13)?

_____

_____

_____

What does Jesus's request to "give us today our daily bread" (verse 11) tell us about the way God provides for our needs?

_____

_____

_____

What did Jesus mean when He said, "lead us not into temptation" (verse 13)?

_____

_____

_____

Why do you think Jesus included each of these particular requests?

_____

_____

_____

The brevity of the Lord's Prayer has many implications for us as praying people. First, we do not need to impress God with the number of our words or the quality of our speech. Poetic, flowery speech is unnecessary; our natural yet respectful language is enough to convey what is on our hearts. Actually, the very words themselves are not as important, for God knows what we need before we even ask (see Matthew 6:8). What's most important is that we have come God in the first place with our adoration and concerns. In light of Christ's teaching about keeping our prayers simple, write a prayer that expresses what is on your heart. Begin with a sentence of adoration and then be specific about how you would like the Lord to work in your life.

_____

_____

_____

Lord, thank You that I can be myself as I come to You each day. Thank You for the example Jesus left for us on how pray. Nudge me, Father, so I am with You all day long. In Jesus's name, amen.

—— DAY 3: PRAY SINCERELY

Lord, I want to pray on a consistent basis, but life gets hectic and it is hard to have uninterrupted time. Guide me so I can hear from You on a more disciplined basis. In Jesus's name, amen.

Those who practice the spiritual exercise of prayerwalking might wrestle with mentioning it publicly. Although they know the practice helps them physically, emotionally, and spiritually, they may not want to flaunt their devotional practices in front of their neighbors, for to do so seems contrary to Jesus's teaching in Matthew 6:1-6, 16-18.[1] Read those verses now. What three different acts of righteousness does Jesus discuss (see verses 2, 5, 16)?

_____

_____

_____

What do you think ties those three faith practices together?

_____

_____

_____

Jesus taught that those who seek the praise of humans rather than God are hypocrites. When these people pray, they are not truly seeking God's help for their lives but only want to be viewed as important and spiritual in the eyes of others. Hypocrites' reward is human praise—not God's direction. Where does Jesus teach we should pray (see verse 6)?

_____

_____

_____

And how should we pray (see verse 6)?

_____

_____

_____

Why would Jesus teach us to pray away from the attention of others?

_____

_____

_____

You don't have to make a big deal out of your devotional time, and you don't have to flaunt it in front of others. Instead, you can pray quietly and sincerely. While you can always pray silently on-the-go for needs as they arise, it is also important to spend dedicated time with God for your family members' and friends' needs, the tasks you have ahead, and the burdens that weigh on your heart. For this quiet time with God, you want to set aside a time and place where you won't be interrupted. One woman goes to her prayer chair in the early morning—just a comfy chair in the corner of her living room. Others keep a journal at their bedside and pray before they go to sleep. One young mom says she prays in her bathroom—and her six children, ages two to nine, have strict instructions about leaving mommy alone when she is in her "prayer closet." Where will be the best time and place for you to pray?

_____

_____

_____

If this is a new devotional practice for you, when will you start?

_____

_____

_____

Father, I am excited about our appointment in prayer and thank You that You care enough about me to want to hear what is on my heart. In Jesus's name, amen.

—— DAY 4: PRAY PERSISTENTLY

Lord, thank You for persevering in pursuing a relationship with me and teaching me to be perseverant in prayer as well. In Jesus' name, amen.

One of the most important characteristics we can develop is perseverance. Schoolteachers know the brightest students are not always the most successful, because they rely on their brainpower to ace tests or do work more quickly than others. When those students are faced with more difficult material in college, they often falter because they are not used to reading textbooks, taking notes, or studying for exams. On the other hand, students who turn in every assignment on time and work at mastering the material tend to find success in college. This is true because they have developed the quality of perseverance—that characteristic of being devoted to their studies in spite of challenges. Read Luke 18:1-8. In this parable on prayer, what did the widow want from the judge (see verse 3)?

_____

_____

_____

What was the judge's initial response to her request (see verse 4)?

_____

_____

_____

What did the judge finally decide to do (see verses 4-5)?

_____

_____

_____

Why do you think the judge changed his mind?

_____

_____

_____

How are God's people described in verse 7?

_____

_____

_____

How will God respond to those who cry out to Him day and night (see verse 8)?

_____

_____

_____

The judge in this parable did not fear God or care about people, and Jesus even called him "unjust." Nonetheless, because the widow pleaded her case with him at every opportunity, he gave in and ruled in her favor. We, however, have a just God who loves to meet our needs. In fact, we have an advantage with God. You have probably heard people say the older a couple gets, the more they look and act like each other. The same is true for those who believe. The more time we spend in prayer and in studying God's Word, the more our character resembles that of Christ. Prayer puts us into another realm—the spiritual realm. As we become more aware of God and even like-minded with Him, He bends our hearts and minds toward His. As we persevere in prayer, we can expect our just God to answer in just the right time. Think about your biggest prayer needs right now. Which ones may require persistent prayer?

_____

_____

_____

If these needs are big, important, and life-changing, they are worthy of your time in prayer. So in the days, weeks, and months ahead, demonstrate to God their importance to you and keep going back to the Judge. At your next First Place for Health meeting, consider sharing these concerns on your Prayer Partner sheet so someone else can join in and support you in this way.

Dear Father, it is my desire to develop the quality of perseverance in my life. I want to pray regularly, and as I do that, to be persistent in lifting up the burdens of my heart. Thank You for being a just God who wants the best for me. In Jesus's name, amen.

—— DAY 5: PRAY BOLDLY

Lord, sometimes I feel like a street corner beggar asking for a handout all the time. Help me to approach You confidently and boldly with my requests. In Jesus's name, amen.

In *The Circle Maker* Mark Batterson writes, "If your prayers aren't impossible to you, they are insulting to God. Why? Because they don't require divine intervention. But ask God to part the Red Sea or make the sun stand still or float an iron axhead, and God is moved to omnipotent action. . . . The greatest moments in life are the miraculous moments when human impotence and divine omnipotence intersect—and they intersect when we draw a circle around the impossible situations in our lives and ask God to intervene."[2] Thankfully, we serve a God who not only knows how to give us good gifts but also delights in blessing us. Read Luke 11:5-13. What is the friend's problem? What bold action does he take to solve it (see verses 5-6)?

_____

_____

_____

What is the neighbor's initial reaction (see verse 7)? Why?

_____

_____

_____

Why does the neighbor change his mind (see verse 8)?

_____

_____

_____

What principle about prayer does Jesus give us in verses 9-10? How should we pray in light of these teachings?

_____

_____

_____

According to verses 11-13, what kind of gifts does our heavenly Father like to give us?

_____

_____

_____

God honors our bold prayers. This is not to say we should have a name-it-and-claim-it mentality. God certainly wants to prosper us, but He is most concerned with the condition of our hearts. On the other hand, if we only pray for things we know we can get easily, there is not a lot of honor there for God. Instead, Jesus urges us to pray big, bold, impossible prayers—prayers that are beyond our reach. These are prayers that, when answered, make us say, "God did this! I give Him all the credit!" What is at least one bold request you will make to God?

_____

_____

_____

Lord, it is exciting that You love to hear my bold prayers. Thank You for giving good gifts. I am so grateful that I worship and serve a God who does the impossible. In Jesus's name, amen.

—— DAY 6: REFLECTION AND APPLICATION

Lord, my coming to You in prayer is a statement of faith, but at times I feel as though my faith is so small. Increase my faith day by day as I see You working in my life. In Jesus's name, amen.

In Mark 9:14-29 we read that as Jesus and His disciples were approaching a crowd, a man came up to them and begged Jesus to heal his son who was suffering from seizures. Jesus asked how long the boy had been suffering, and the father replied since childhood. Then he said, "But if you can do anything, take pity on us and help us."

Jesus said, "'If you can'? Everything is possible for one who believes" (verse 23). The father immediately exclaimed, "I do believe; help me overcome my unbelief" (verse 24).

Jesus then rebuked the demon who had been tormenting the boy and healed him. This puzzled the disciples because they had unsuccessfully tried to heal the boy themselves. They asked Jesus why they couldn't drive out the demon.

Jesus replied, "This kind can come out only by prayer" (verse 29).

In the parallel account told in Matthew 17:14-23, Jesus then related the well-known mustard seed metaphor: "Truly I tell you, if you have faith as small as a mustard seed, you can say to this mountain, 'Move from here to there' and it will move. Nothing will be impossible for you" (verse 20).

Through prayer we partner with God in faith to do the impossible. Our faith need not match the size of the prayer. Our faith need not be as big as the miracle-to-be. Simply going to the Father with our requests—large or small—is an act of faith.

The father of the boy in the story said he believed, but he asked Christ to help him with his unbelief. Our faith is imperfect, and our prayers may be imperfect, but as we partner with our perfect God in prayer for the work of the impossible, He will increase our faith. Ole Hallesby, a little known but powerful author on prayer, once wrote, "The essence of faith is to come to Christ. . . . It is not intended that our faith should help Jesus to fulfill our supplications. He does not need any help; all He needs is access. Neither is it intended that our faith should draw Jesus into our distress, or make Him interested in us, or solicitous on our behalf. But He can not gain admittance until we 'open the door'."[3]

What is incredible about prayer is that Christ initiated the conversation with us. He said, "Here I am! I stand at the door and knock. If anyone hears my voice and opens the door, I will come in and eat with that person, and they with me" (Revelation 3:20). He merely needs us to open the door of our hearts so as to continue that lifelong conversation.

Lord, thank You for seeking out a relationship with me. It is so incredible that I can partner with the God of the universe in pursuit of the impossible. I look forward to seeing how You will grow my faith through prayer. In Jesus's name, amen.

—— DAY 7: REFLECTION AND APPLICATION

Father, thank You for sending Your Son, Jesus, to provide a way for me to have a relationship with You. Thank You that as He walked on this earth, He taught us how to be bold and persistent in our prayers. In Jesus's name, amen.

Prayer is important to our devotional life, but it is just one facet. Studying God's Word is also essential, as it can transform our thinking and desires. Reading the Bible on a daily basis breathes spiritual life into our heart, mind, and soul. As our thinking changes to align more closely with biblical truth, our prayers also become like-minded with God's plan.

It is not always easy to pray in the Father's will. We can certainly see that in the life of Jesus when He faced the cross. In the Garden of Gethsemane, He prayed, "My Father, if it is possible, may this cup be taken from me. Yet not as I will, but as you will" (Matthew 26:39). This simple prayer shows us that we can approach God with our human heart's desire and yet also pray for God's will to be done. This is a two-sided-coin prayer. One side is what we long for, while the other is what God knows is best.

This kind of prayer may be the best and most honest one we can give. Even so, we know that God accepts such a prayer because He accepted it from His Son. And just as Jesus became an instrument of God by praying that prayer, we can as well. Our two-sided-coin prayer may be our best attempt at a holy act: "Lord, Your will be done."

We may never know why some prayers are answered and some are not. But by studying God's Word and faithfully going to Him in prayer, our natures and our will can be gradually bent to His, step-by-step, day-by-day, decision-by-decision. As

Herbert Lockyer wrote, "The whole purpose of prayer is the accomplishment of his known will."[4] Whatever the results and answers are, prayer can bring about God's will in our lives.

As you continue in your First Place for Health journey, what are your greatest desires in the following four areas that you will commit to prayer?

Physical

_____
_____
_____

Mental

_____
_____
_____

Emotional

_____
_____
_____

Spiritual

_____
_____
_____

Keep in mind that God can do the impossible through you as you partner with Him in prayer!

Lord of my heart, I give to You all these areas of my life. I already sense that You are working through me, and I look forward to partnering with You in prayer. I truly believe You are a God of the impossible! In Jesus's name, amen.

Notes

1. Janet Holm McHenry, *PrayerWalk* (Colorado Springs, CO: WaterBrook, 2011).

2. Mark Batterson, *The Circle Maker* (Grand Rapids, MI: Zondervan, 2011), 13.

3. Ole Hallesby, *Prayer* (Minneapolis, MN: Augsburg, 1994), 30-31.

4. Herbert Lockyer, *All the Prayers of the Bible* (Grand Rapids, MI: Zondervan, 1959), 272.

WEEK TWO: TRAINING IN FORGIVENESS

SCRIPTURE MEMORY VERSE
Bear with each other and forgive whatever grievances you may have against one another. Forgive as the Lord forgave you. Colossians 3:13

In Acts 6:1-7 we read that the number of believers in the early church was growing so rapidly that the disciples needed to recruit seven more leaders to attend to ministry matters. Among them was Stephen, a man full of God's grace and power, who performed many miracles. Because of Stephen's effectiveness in ministry, those in opposition began telling lies about him to try to discredit him. Eventually, he was brought before the Sanhedrin—the highest council—where false witnesses testified against him.

The high priest then asked Stephen, "Are these charges true?" (Acts 7:1). Stephen answered by recalling the history of how God had pursued His people over the generations, culminating with His gift of the "Righteous One," Jesus Christ. The members of the Sanhedrin were so outraged at Stephen's testimony that they dragged him out of the city and stoned him.

Stephen would die from the blows, but before he did, he said, "Lord, do not hold this sin against them" (verse 60). Stephen was able to forgive his murderers because of Christ's teaching on forgiveness and how He demonstrated that quality in His life. However, this trait does not develop automatically as we embrace the Christian faith.

When others hurt us, it is natural for us to want to simmer in resentment, spurt out in anger, or stew in bitterness. When we feel wronged, an in-born streak of justice flames up in us and makes us burn. When we feel helpless to do anything about the situation, we might even seek out the sympathy of others—and in this way spread the offense so it creates division among friends, co-workers, or family members. We might even pray, "God, do something!"

But God did, in fact, do something. He sent His Son so that we might not only hear and witness Christ's teachings about forgiveness but also experience it for ourselves. God gave Jesus, our Personal Trainer, a mission to bring forgiveness to us. As we become more forgiving people, others will be drawn to Him.

—— DAY 1: FORGIVE DEBTS

Lord, it is often hard to discern how I should respond when others hurt me. Help me to understand about how to react when life is not fair. In Jesus's name, amen.

Last week we studied the Lord's Prayer. Reread Matthew 6:12, the final portion of Jesus's prayer that addresses forgiveness. Some translations use the word debts in that verse, some use sins, and some use trespasses. How would you define each of those words?

_____

_____

_____

Recall a time when someone hurt you. What was the situation? How did it make you feel?

_____

_____

_____

How do you think the other person felt? How did the offense affect your relationship?

_____

_____

_____

Read Jesus's follow-up teaching in Matthew 6:14-15. What happens when we forgive others?

_____

_____

_____

What happens when we do not forgive others?

_____

_____

_____

Offenses can create a crack in a relationship, but the lack of forgiveness can cause a permanent break. A right relationship with others is important if we expect to have a right relationship with God. What are three earthly consequences that could occur as a result of a lack of forgiveness?

_____

_____

_____

Think of a few people right now you need to forgive. Ask God to help you forgive them and remove the power of their offense, and then thank God for forgiving you of your debts, sins, and trespasses. Conclude by thanking Him for how your acts of forgiveness will free you of resentment, anger, and bitterness.

Lord, I am grateful that You have forgiven me. With Your help, I will choose to be more Christ-like by forgiving others before the hurt manifests in ugly ways. In Jesus's name, amen.

——— DAY 2: BE RECONCILED

Lord, how it must hurt You when Your children have conflicts with each other. Prompt me, Lord, when I have wronged someone so I do not create division in Your family. In Jesus's name, amen.

There are two sides of the record album of forgiveness. On the one side we need to forgive others when they wrong us, but on the flip side, we must also seek others' forgiveness when we have hurt them. Read Matthew 5:23-26. How would you summarize this passage?

_____

_____

_____

Jesus teaches that we should not make an offering to God if we have a broken relationship with someone. Why would our offering not be acceptable in such cases?

_____

_____

_____

In Jesus's day, some people gave money as an offering (see Luke 21:1-2), while others might have given an animal from their flock (see Leviticus 1:3), and travelers might have purchased cattle, sheep, or doves (see John 2:14). If someone had to leave the gift to seek another's forgiveness, what could happen to the gift? How might that person feel about leaving an offering?

_____

_____

_____

When I taught high school English, I gave this formula to my students on how to ask forgiveness: "I was wrong when I _____. Will you forgive me?" When we have to admit the actual offense and then ask for forgiveness, it makes us think twice about doing the same thing again. Using this language helps bring about restoration more fully than a simple "sorry." Also, if the offense occurred publicly, the apology should be made in front of the same people—or at least communicated to the others if the setting cannot be similarly staged.

One day, a student in my class insulted me, and I reacted emotionally with a sarcastic remark. Naturally, the student lashed out even more, and I had a mess on my hands. The next day I told my class, "I was wrong when I insulted 'George' yesterday. I should not have reacted the way I did. Will you forgive me, George?" The student immediately said "yes" and owned up to his own inappropriate language. Life with George was just fine after that day.

It is true that some cases might require restitution before forgiveness can be fully granted. For example, if you borrowed your neighbor's lawn mower and broke the starter cord, it would be appropriate not only to apologize but also to get the mower fixed or even purchase a new one for your neighbor. Reread Matthew 5:25-26. Why does Jesus emphasize that restoration with an adversary happen quickly?

_____

_____

_____

Sometimes we sense tension in a relationship with another person. Even if we are not sure of the offense, we can approach that person to re-establish communication. That conversation could start like this: "I sense there's some distance between us, and if I have done something to offend or hurt you, I would like to know, because I value our relationship." Do you need to apologize to someone? If so, complete this chart, make a commitment as to when you will make a phone call or a personal visit (an electronic message is not appropriate for this type of communication), and pray that God will give you the right words.

What the offense is	
Date I will contact that person	
What I will say	

Lord, thank You for giving me many chances when I make mistakes. I ask for Your grace to cover me as I keep my relationships clean by asking forgiveness of others. In Jesus's name, amen.

—— DAY 3: FORGIVE CONTINUALLY

Father, it is difficult to forgive time after time. Remind me daily of the graces and mercies You show to me so that forgiveness becomes second nature in my character. In Jesus's name, amen.

We believe in continuous grace and merciful forgiveness—when we are on the receiving end. But we can weary quickly when others hurt us again and again. Jesus told a story that deals with this very issue in Matthew 18:21-35. What question did Peter ask that prompted Jesus to tell this parable (see verse 21)?

_____

_____

_____

Why do you think Peter asked this question?

_____

_____

_____

Jewish tradition taught that a person must forgive three times but not four. Peter probably expected Jesus to be twice as generous, so he more than doubled the number when he asked, "Up to seven times?" (verse 21). How did Jesus respond (see verse 22)?

_____

_____

_____

Some versions of the Bible say "seventy times seven" instead of "seventy-seven times." The point is that Jesus does not lay out a fixed number of times we must forgive and then check off when someone offends us. We do not count offenses legalistically for the reason He describes in parable that follows. Complete the following chart for the two parts of the story.

	King and the Servant	*Servant and Fellow Servant*
How much is owed?	*v. 24:*	*v. 28:*
How does the person owed the money respond?	*v. 25:*	*v. 28:*
How does the debtor respond?	*v. 26:*	*v. 29:*
How does the person owed then respond?	*v. 27:*	*v. 30:*

What characteristics does the king demonstrate toward his servant?

_____

_____

_____

What characteristics does the servant demonstrate toward his fellow servant?

_____

_____

_____

In the parable Jesus includes onlookers who have observed the unmerciful behavior of the first servant. The servant owed the king 10,000 talents; one single talent is believed to be the equivalent of roughly 16 years' wages. The fellow servant owed the servant 100 denarii; one denarius was worth the equivalent of a day's wage.[1] It is no surprise, then, that the onlookers let the king know of his servant's lack of mercy—and that the king changed his mind and had the first servant punished until his debt was paid.

Thankfully, when we profess our faith in Christ, we are forgiven forever. In Romans 8:1 Paul wrote, "Therefore, there is now no condemnation for those who are in Christ Jesus." However, as forgiven people we should demonstrate God's great grace and mercy by forgiving others—not just seven times, or 77 times, but an infinite number. That does not mean we permit people to abuse or damage us or those we love, but as we make others accountable for their actions, we still forgive them in our hearts.

Lord, thank You for forgiving me once and for all time to come. Keep my heart soft so that Your love fills me and compels me to demonstrate Your forgiving nature. In Jesus's name, amen.

—— DAY 4: LET IT GO
Lord, I know I should forgive, but judgment and anger still seem to ruminate inside of me. Help me to let go so I am free of the offense. In Jesus's name, amen.

We all have heard the expression forgive and forget. We have also heard people say, "I'll forgive him, but I won't forget what he did." Unfortunately, we may be some of those people. I recently found myself holding on to a grudge against someone—until my three-year-old granddaughter, Temperance, taught me a lesson.

Tempe, her five siblings, and I were on my living room couch watching the movie Frozen. When the character Elsa started to sing "Let It Go," Tempe spun in circles, arms poised heavenward, and sang, "Wet it go, wet it go!"

I laughed, but then it struck me: "Wet it go, Janet!" I determined to not only forgive the offender but also also refuse to take offense. So, I "wet it go," and now I often sing those memorable lines from the song to remind myself that I can choose my attitudes toward others.

Forgive and forget may not be a biblical expression, but it is a principle that Jesus demonstrates. Complete the following chart:

Verse(s)	Name of person	What did this person do to Jesus?
Luke 22:47-48		
Luke 22:60-61		
Luke 22:63		
Luke 23:11		
Luke 23:21		
Luke 23:33		

Despite the betrayal, denial, beatings, mocking, and crucifixion, what did Jesus pray in Luke 23:34?

_____

_____

_____

In other words, Jesus said, "Let it go." He not only forgave, but He also asked His heavenly Father to forgive those who hurt Him. Refusing to forget—allowing judgment and condemnation to linger—is an indication that we have not yet trusted God to deal with the offender and take care of the consequences. In the process of reliving the incident, we allow it to injure us again and again, allowing anger, resentment, and even bitterness to paralyze our memory and cripple our present.

When the other person seeks reconciliation and forgiveness and we refuse, we are the ones now impeding a relationship—with that person and with God. When we harbor anger and resentment, we continue to allow that person to have control over us. It is just not a healthy situation, and any refusal to let it go could impede our participation in God's greater plan for for that situation and for our life. With that in mind, if someone's offense still bothers you, write your prayer below to let it go.

_____

_____

_____

Now blacken it with a marker. It's not erased, but it is covered over. Allow God to deal with the details of restoration as you choose to let it go.

Lord, thank You for inspiring me to be free of judgment and condemnation as I choose to let go of any unforgiveness I have harbored toward others. In Jesus's name, amen.

—— DAY 5: EMPATHIZE

Father, help me to put myself in the other person's shoes so that I better understand the pain and frustrations that he or she feels. In Jesus's name, amen.

Jesus gave us another example of forgiveness when He was hanging on the cross. Read the full account in Luke 23:26-43. As you read about His walking toward the location of the crucifixion, how can you know that Jesus did not feel sorry for Himself (see verses 27-28)?

_____

_____

_____

Jesus and two criminals were executed in a manner that was meant to be painful and prolonged. What did one of the criminals say to Jesus in verse 39? But how did the second criminal respond (see verses 40-42)?

_____

_____

_____

Jesus empathized with the men hanging on the crosses next to Him. To the one who offered an insult, He did not respond. How did He respond to the other criminal (see verse 43)? What does Jesus's response imply?

_____

_____

_____

Jesus could offer eternal life to the criminal who believed because He was dying on the cross for him. His empathy for *all* who would believe led Him to the cross of forgiveness. The Greek root of the word *empathy* offers the sense that a person suffers with another and tries to understand that person's feelings. It was Jesus's suffering for others that made Him suffer for their sake.

In Harper Lee's novel *To Kill a Mockingbird*, set in a small Alabama town during the 1930s, Atticus Finch teaches his two children, Scout and Jem, by words and example. One of his iconic lines is, "You never really understand a person until you consider things from his point of view . . . until you climb into his skin and walk around in it." As the children grow up, they have plenty of opportunities to empathize with the neighbors around them—hypocritical missionary circle ladies, white racists, mean neighbors, the mentally ill, and African-Americans. When Scout finally meets the elusive Boo Radley and realizes he is kind and even heroic, Atticus says, "Most people are, Scout, when you finally see them."[2]

If we want to be more like our Personal Trainer, we need to ask the Lord to help us really see other people—to help us understand and even empathize with their life situation and the challenges they face. In the space below, write the name of a person you have struggled with in the past. Then write down some of the hardships that person might be facing.

_____

_____

_____

Pray for an opportunity to express your empathy in a practical way to that person—through a note, gift, meal, or other kindness that could lighten that person's load.

Lord, Your mercies never fail but continue to flow like an unquenchable mountain stream. Help me to put myself in the shoes of others so I understand their position before I lash back out of hurt. In Jesus's name, amen.

—— DAY 6: REFLECTION AND APPLICATION
Father, thank You for sending Your Son, Jesus, for the forgiveness of my sins. Because of Your gift, I can freely forgive as well. In Jesus's name, amen.

In this week's Scripture memory verse Paul tells us we are to forgive as the Lord forgave us (see Colossians 3:13). The whole concept of forgiveness, then, is not just a requirement but also a God-given gift as exemplified through His Son, Jesus.

In Matthew 26:26-28 we read about the Last Supper that Jesus had with His disciples before His crucifixion. This passage tells us that while they were eating, Jesus took bread, gave thanks for it, broke the bread, and gave it to His disciples, saying, "Take and eat; this is my body" (verse 26). Then he took a cup of what we would assume was wine, gave thanks for it, and gave it to them, saying, "Drink from it, all of you. This is my blood of the covenant, which is poured out for many for the forgiveness of sins" (verses 27-28).

The bread and wine were symbols for Jesus's body and His blood. Those food objects foreshadowed the giving of His life for the forgiveness of sins from that point forward. In other words, He gave His life for the sake of forgiveness.

We also give up something when we forgive others. It could be our anger, our bitterness, our pride, or our hurt. Complete forgiveness might also require us to give up a pattern of complaining or gossiping or making excuses for our behavior. On the other hand forgiveness releases us from mental, emotional, and spiritual chains that tie us down to baggage that would keep us from living freely. It allows peace and contentment to reign in our demeanor and in our relationships with others.

How could forgiveness—the acceptance of it and the gift of it to others—allow you to live more freely in the following areas of your life?

Physical

_____
_____
_____

Mental

_____
_____
_____

Emotional

_____
_____
_____

Spiritual

_____
_____
_____

Lord, thank You for the gift of Your life for the forgiveness of my sins. Prod me to give of myself for the sake of healthy relationships as I attempt to follow Your example. In Jesus's name, amen.

—— DAY 7: REFLECTION AND APPLICATION
Father, sometimes the person I need to forgive is myself. Thank You that Your cross is like a cancellation "X" that crosses out my mistakes. In Jesus's name, amen.

Missionary and scholar David Seamands wrote, "There is no forgiveness from God unless you freely forgive your brother from your heart. And I wonder if we have been too narrow in thinking that 'brother' only applies to someone else. What if YOU are the brother or sister who needs to be forgiven, and you need to forgive yourself?"[3] If you have been holding on to a past sin in your life, here is a process for how you can forgive yourself:

1. **Confess it**. "If we confess our sins, he is faithful and just and will forgive us our sins and purify us from all unrighteousness" (1 John 1:9). If something is weighing on you, confess it now to God.
2. **Make amends.** "Go and be reconciled to your brother" (Matthew 5:24). If someone else is involved, make your sincere apology to that person and also make any needed restitution.
3. **Stop wallowing in it.** "The LORD our God said . . . 'You have stayed long enough at this mountain'" (Deuteronomy 1:6). Decide to move past this mountain of guilt that has paralyzed you and kept you from living freely.
4. **Choose positivity as an attitude.** "Finally, brothers and sisters, whatever is true, whatever is noble, whatever is right, whatever is pure, whatever is lovely, whatever is admirable—if anything is excellent or praiseworthy—think about such things" (Philippians 4:8). Let the past be the past. Decide to focus on the good traits and blessings God has given you so that others around you see your new, positive outlook.
5. **Learn from it.** "Not that I have already obtained all this, or have already arrived at my goal, but I press on to take hold of that for which Christ Jesus took hold of me" (Philippians 3:12). Determine to make better choices so that the past has purpose and the present is positive.
6. **Shift to an outward focus.** "I am coming to you now, but I say these things while I am still in the world, so that they may have the full measure of my joy within them" (John 17:13). Live for the purpose of bringing others joy.

Write a prayer of forgiveness: Lord, I forgive myself for . . .

_____

_____

_____

_____

_____

_____

_____

Notes

1. Mary Fairchild, "What Is a Talent," About Religion, accessed November 21, 2015, http://christianity.about.com/od/glossary/a/Talent.htm.

2. Harper Lee, To Kill a Mockingbird (New York: HarperCollins, 1960).

3. David Seamands, Healing for Damaged Emotions (Wheaton, IL: Victor Books, 1981), 31-32.

WEEK THREE: TRAINING IN DETERMINATION

SCRIPTURE MEMORY VERSE
I can do all this through him who gives me strength. Philippians 4:13

Olympic gold medalist Wilma Rudolph was an inspiration to many because of her determination to overcome her handicaps and be a world athlete. Born prematurely in 1940, she weighed just four and a half pounds and spent much of her childhood in bed due to double pneumonia, scarlet fever, and polio. She wore metal leg braces starting at age six but said, "I spent most of my time trying to figure out how to get them off."[1]

She grew up poor—the sixteenth of her father's nineteen children from two marriages. Her father was a railroad porter, and her mother was a domestic worker.[2] One day she asked her parents, "Will I ever be able to run and play like the other children?" They told her that if she believed in God and never gave up hope, He would make it happen.[3]

He did. By the time she was 11, she stunned her doctors by walking without her leg braces. "By the time I was 12," she told the *Chicago Tribune*, "I was challenging every boy in our neighborhood at running, jumping, everything."

With her own determination and the efforts of her devoted family—her siblings massaged her legs daily and her mother drove her 90 miles round-trip to physical therapy—she overcame her disability and won four Olympic medals: a bronze medal in the 1956 4x100 relay and three gold medals in 1960 in the 4x100 relay, the 100m, and the 200m.[4]

—— DAY 1: GET FOCUSED

Father, just as Your Son was determined to live out His life on earth for the calling on His life, I also want to be focused on the path You have for me. In Jesus's name, amen.

Jesus lived out His life with purpose. His daily tasks—teaching, healing the masses, answering questions from religious leaders—were all part of His walk toward the Calvary cross. All those days on earth culminated in His greatest accomplishment: offering Himself as a sacrifice to atone for the sins of humankind for all time. Through His death He provided a way for those who believe in Him to have eternal life.

Even from a young age Jesus focus on His heavenly Father's calling. When He was 12, His family traveled to Jerusalem to celebrate Passover and He went missing for three days. The story in Luke 2:41-52 tells us that His parents found Him in the Temple courts listening to the teachers and asking them questions. Those who heard Him were "amazed at his understanding and his answers" (verse 47). When his mother asked why He had treated them with such disregard, He said, "Didn't you know I had to be in my Father's house?" (verse 49). The adolescent who would become the Savior was already focused on His calling.

Throughout the Gospel of John, Jesus uses "I am" statements to tell His listeners about Himself—about what was His purpose on earth. Look up each of the verses in the chart below and write what Jesus called Himself. Then explain in your own words what you think He meant.

	What Jesus called Himself	What this Means
John 6:35, 41, 51		
John 8:12		
John 10:7, 9		
John 10:11, 14		
John 10:36		

Based on these "I am" statements, what do you think Jesus's purpose was on earth?

_____

_____

_____

Jesus knew who He was: God's only Son who came to earth so others could know the Lord God, have a personal relationship with Him, and have eternal life. How would you define who you are (daughter, sister, teacher, ministry leader, volunteer)?

_____

_____

_____

A calling is a divinely inspired purpose or direction for life. This could be an occupation, ministry, career, or avocation of some type. Often the calling will relate to natural talents and interests you have. What is your purpose or calling? (If you are not sure, take some time to ask God to speak to your heart. He will always answer when we pray, "Here I am, Lord! Send me!")

_____

_____

_____

Lord, I am excited that You have a purpose for my life! Teach me and guide me in Your calling. May the rest of my days bring You joy as I determine to follow You. In Jesus's name, amen.

—— DAY 2: SET PRIORITIES

Father, I know You have a calling on my life, but sometimes the urgent stomps all over the important. Help me set priorities so my life is purposeful. In Jesus's name, amen.

In 1896 minister Charles Sheldon published the novel *In His Steps: What Would Jesus Do?* As the story opens, Reverend Maxwell, the main character, is struggling on a Friday to finish his Sunday sermon, the focus of which is 1 Peter 2:21: "To this you were called, because Christ suffered for you, leaving you an example, that you should follow in his steps." Interruptions had been a problem, and to make matters worse, a shabby man comes to the door asking for leads on jobs in the area. The minister says he knows of nothing and shuts the door.

The preacher pulls the sermon together to his satisfaction. Two days later, just after he delivers it with great effect to his congregation, the same shabby man appears in front of the pulpit with a message of his own. New machines had put the printer out of work 10 months ago, his wife had died four months ago, and his little girl was staying with another family. He had tramped across the country looking for work—the last three days in Maxwell's town. "In all that time," he says, "I've not had a word of sympathy or comfort except from your minister here, who said he was sorry for me and hoped I would find a job somewhere."

As the man recounts the difficulties he and his family have experienced, he has one question for the Christian congregation: *What does following Jesus mean?* The rest of the novel chronicles how the people of the town responded to that question: *What would Jesus do?* As we look at the Gospels, we see that what Jesus did was focus His life on several priorities: His relationship with His Father, people, the teaching of truth, and obedience.

Read Mark 12:28-31. What are the two parts of the greatest commandment?

_____

_____

_____

Christ made communicating with His heavenly Father a priority, but He also valued people and made their needs a priority. How do you prioritize people's needs in your life?

_____

_____

_____

Jesus also prioritized teaching the truth. In fact, if He had a motto, it could have been "I tell you the truth," because the Gospels record numerous examples of His saying this—at least 30 in Matthew alone. Read Matthew 24:34-35. What does Jesus say? How has this been proven true?

_____

_____

_____

Jesus also prioritized obedience to the Father. Read Philippians 2:8. How did Jesus demonstrate His obedience to His calling?

_____

_____

_____

What are your priorities? Make a list of them, starting with the most important. Now give them to God in prayer and see how He leads you in the days ahead.

_____

_____

_____

Father God, thank You for the example of Your Son, who determined to love You fully, help others faithfully, teach people truthfully, and obey You completely. In Jesus's name, amen.

—— DAY 3: PERSEVERE

Lord, life isn't easy, and some days I want to pull the covers over my head and go back to sleep. Instead, show me the value of working hard and persevering. In Jesus's name, amen.

Once you have set a new course for your life physically, mentally, emotionally, and spiritually, you will inevitably encounter hardships that will waylay you. You might get injured or sick. Someone in your family might lose a job. Such tough circumstances can easily become excuses to make you want to quit. Read Luke 5:17-26. When the friends of the paralytic cannot get through the crowd to Jesus, what do they do (verse 19)?

_____

_____

_____

In what two ways does Jesus respond (see verses 20, 24)?

_____

_____

_____

What would have been the result for the crippled man if his friends had given up?

_____

_____

_____

What situation has seemingly crippled your attempts to get stronger and healthier through the First Place for Health program?

_____

_____

_____

How could your group members help you through this roadblock?

_____

_____

_____

What steps could you take to overcome any challenges you may be facing right now?

_____

_____

_____

Lord, help me to overcome any paralysis in progress that would otherwise keep me from getting stronger and healthier. In Jesus's name, amen.

—— DAY 4: AVOID PROCRASTINATION

Lord, I am thankful that You have entrusted me with gifts and talents. Help me to avoid procrastination so that my days honor You. In Jesus's name, amen.

A funny sign outside a meeting hall read, "Today's Procrastinators Anonymous meeting has been changed to tomorrow."

There are lots of reasons for procrastinating. According to researchers at the University of North Carolina, some people procrastinate because they are afraid. They fear that failure or, oddly, even success might increase others' expectations of them. Some fear a loss of autonomy and so passively reject whatever someone asks them to do. Depending on the task, others fear being alone if a connection with others would end, or they fear becoming attached if the task requires working with others.

Other reasons for procrastination include a need for perfection. Perfectionists often put off a task because they know they do not have enough time to get it done in the exact way they want. Another reason is that the task simply is not enjoyable—so procrastination is avoidance of displeasure. Additionally, people might put things off if they are too busy or if they know others will do the work for them if they delay.[5] Read Luke 9:59-62. When Jesus invites the first man to follow Him, how does he reply (see verse 59)?

_____
_____
_____

What is Jesus's response (see verse 60)?

_____
_____
_____

How does the second man respond to Jesus's invitation to follow Him (see verse 61)?

_____
_____
_____

What is Jesus's response to this man (see verse 62)?

_____
_____
_____

While Jesus's responses may seem harsh, His time on earth was limited so he needed those who were determined, focused, and committed to His ministry. The first man would have already been with his family if his father was dead—he was just making excuses and delaying action. Jesus's response to the second man also acknowledged an excuse. Looking backward while plowing would create uneven rows and get the farmer completely off course. So, too, our reasons and excuses of procrastination get us off course. Here are some suggestions to overcome procrastination:

1. **Write down your daily tasks** on a to-do list and plan when during your day you will complete each one.
2. **Determine not to delay action**, and then check off those items. If you don't, the items will compound for the next day's to-do list, and those tasks will only create more stress for you.

3. **Let go of perfectionistic tendencies.** A job completed well is certainly better than one not even attempted.
4. **Exercise daily** so you are energized for the tasks ahead.
5. Simplify your life. Clear your life, schedule, and home of the things you know bog you down and require your attention.
6. **Study your Bible** and pray daily so you have clear direction from God about what is important and what is not.
7. **Get good sleep** so you are refreshed each morning for the day ahead.

Proverbs 27:1 says, "Do not boast about tomorrow, for you do not know what a day may bring." Today is an opportunity to shine, so make the most of it!

Father, help me to make the most of my day so that at the end of it I can sense Your smile on me. In Jesus's name, amen.

—— DAY 5: FEND OFF DISTRACTIONS

Father, there are so many distractions today with so many demands calling my name. Teach me how to avoid distraction so I am productive. In Jesus's name, amen.

There are many electronics calling our name these days. Television. Social media. Videos. Online retail websites. Email. Phone texts. Any of these can pull us away from our determined course. Read Luke 10:38-42. In this passage Jesus and His disciples travel from Jerusalem to Bethany, about two miles to the east. Who opens her home to Jesus (see verse 38)?

_____

_____

_____

Two sisters live in the home: Martha and Mary. What does Mary do for Jesus, her guest (see verse 39)?

_____

_____

_____

What does Martha do for Jesus, her guest (see verse 40)?

_____

_____

_____

What are Martha's two complaints to Jesus (see verse 40)?

_____

_____

_____

Martha is actually bothered about two people: Mary and Jesus. She is annoyed that Mary is listening to Him, but she is also peeved that Jesus does not notice she is doing all the work—attending to her visitors' needs for cleanliness, arranging liquid refreshments, fixing a meal, and collecting the various utensils to serve the meal. How does Jesus describe Martha (see verse 41)?

_____

_____

_____

Jesus then says, "Few things are needed—or indeed only one. Mary has chosen what is better, and it will not be taken away from her" (verse 42). What is the one thing Mary has chosen? Why would Jesus say the one thing Mary had chosen was better?

_____

_____

_____

Mary is a people person. She takes pleasure in being with others and enjoys their conversation and company. Martha is a doer—her joy comes from completing tasks. However, in this instance, the Lord shows Martha that the most important task at hand is to sit and listen to His teachings and enjoy His presence. All the other tasks are only distractions from that greater task—spending time with Him. What distractions pull you away from what is important?

_____

_____

_____

Notice that Jesus did not complain about Martha's service. She was the one to take her complaint to Him (see verse 40). Also notice that Jesus pulled Martha away from the unimportant—the distractions—to the important by bringing her to Himself. The "one thing" that was needed was that relationship with Him—the conversation, the listening, the presence. Jesus did not dismiss Martha back to the kitchen but drew her to the "one thing"—Himself. How will you handle distractions that you know are pulling you away from what God has purposed for you to do?

_____

_____

_____

Lord, thank You for your graceful nudging that leads me back to You and the course You have set before me. Keep me mindful of the gift of time You have given me. In Jesus's name, amen.

—— DAY 6: REFLECTION AND APPLICATION

Father, when I take on a new goal that honors You, I am bound to face others' criticism. Teach me to recognize when that is not beneficial so I can remain determined. In Jesus's name, amen.

No one likes criticism. We soak in approval, but when others have a critical word, we might withdraw, get defensive, lash out on social media, fall into depression, or even allow the criticism to cause us to quit what we had been doing. However, the example and teachings of our Savior show us how He stayed determined through the never-ending criticism He faced on his road to Calvary.

In the Beatitudes Jesus taught how to respond in the face of criticism: "Blessed are those who are persecuted because of righteousness, for theirs is the kingdom of heaven. Blessed are you when people insult you, persecute you and falsely say all kinds of evil against you because of me. Rejoice and be glad, because great is your reward in heaven, for in the same way they persecuted the prophets who were before you" (Matthew 5:10-12).

While you might not feel blessed when you are being criticized, that not-so-nice comment will allow you to experience a small fraction of the difficulties Christ faced for your sake. Your determination to respond in a godly manner in the throes of criticism will earn rewards for you in heaven. In the meantime, there are always people watching how you will respond, and your reaction to difficulties, pressure, and criticism will do one of two things: attract others to the Christian faith or push them away. You can simply determine to respond in a positive way even when others are being negative.

While correction and reproof are appropriate when we are taking the wrong course, criticism for its own sake can lead us into an emotional mess. Because Jesus is our Personal Trainer, we can examine His life to see how He handled criticism from those who meant to discredit Him. Here is what we find:

1. **He ignored the comment.** When Jesus was called a glutton, a drunkard, and a friend of tax collectors and sinners, He said, "But wisdom is proved right by her deeds" (Matthew 11:19). Despite the critical remarks, Jesus knew His actions would prove His character. Likewise, we can turn our cheek and allow our character to be proven out in time.
2. **He relied on the Word.** Jesus faced several struggles from authorities in regard to His and His disciples' behavior. In Matthew 12:1-8, when Jesus's disciples were gleaning grain to eat from the fields on a Sabbath, He cited incidents from the Old Testament when King David and priests followed the spirit of the law as opposed the letter of the law. While we don't want to fling verses from the Bible around as arrows in a search-and-destroy manner, we can allow the Word to breathe encouragement into our soul and guide us during tough times.
3. **He spoke the truth.** When the Pharisees challenged Jesus about whether it was lawful to heal on the Sabbath, He said, "If any of you has a sheep and it falls into a pit on the Sabbath, will you not take hold of it and lift it out? How much more valuable is a man than a sheep! Therefore it is lawful to do good on the Sabbath" (Matthew 12:11-12). The truth can often dissipate criticism, and calmly stating the truth can bring focus to issues of conflict.

Most likely you have faced some sort of criticism in the past. In light of these glances at the life of your Personal Trainer, how will you respond the next time?

Father, thank You for the example of Your Son, who did not allow His critics to derail Him. Because He bore much for my sake, I can for Him as well. In Jesus's name, amen.

—— DAY 7: REFLECTION AND APPLICATION
Father, I am so blessed that You provide strength for this earthly journey. It is an exciting path, and I am grateful that You are on it with me. In Jesus's name, amen.

In his 1785 ode "To a Mouse," Scotsman Robert Burns wrote, "The best laid schemes o' Mice an' Men gang aft agley, an' lea'e us nought but grief an' pain, for promis'd joy!"[6] This is interpreted in our modern English as, "The best laid schemes of mice and men often go astray, and leave us nothing but grief and pain, for promised joy!"

In the poem, a farmer, who has turned over a mouse's nest with the plough, addresses the mouse, which is all upset because its world has been turned upside down. The farmer sarcastically tells the mouse that it is blessed compared to him, as his past was dreary and his future is filled with fear. While the farmer was exaggerating comically, life simply does not always go as planned. Circumstances occur that we could not have planned or foreseen. They sidetrack us, delay our plans, and stop us in our tracks.

As we determinedly set our gaze on our goals, however, we allow our Personal Trainer to strengthen us so we can have success over circumstances. One way to build inner strength is to meditate on the promises of God's Word, so that when we face challenges, we can draw on our "second wind," just as an athlete would in a race. One way to build Scripture memory is to say the verse aloud many times over, each time emphasizing the next word in the sentence.

Do that now with this week's verse. Say the sentence 10 times, each time emphasizing each successive word: "I can do all this through him who gives me strength" (Philippians 4:13). Then answer these questions:

Who can do everything through Christ who gives strength? _____
What can you do through Christ? _____
Who helps you do everything? _____
What does Christ give you? _____

God's Word is powerful. Allow these words to transform you into a person of confident determination.

Lord, I truly can do everything through You, because You strengthen me for whatever lies ahead. I am so thankful that You are with me every step of my life. In Jesus's name, amen.

Notes

1. M.B. Roberts, "Rudolph Ran and World Went Wild," ESPN.com, accessed September 6, 2015, https://espn.go.com/sportscentury/features/00016444.html.

2. "Wilma Rudolph Biography," Encyclopedia of World Biography, accessed September 6, 2015, http://www.notablebiographies.com/Ro-Sc/Rudolph-Wilma.html.

3. Neil Anderson, "Today's Neil Anderson Devotion," Crosswalk, January 13, 2014, accessed September 6, 2015, http://www.crosswalk.com/devotionals/dailyinchrist/daily-in-christ-1-or-13-544298.html.

4. "Wilma Rudolph." Olympic.org, accessed September 6, 2015, http://www.olympic.org/wilma-rudolph.

5. "Procrastination," The Writing Center, The University of North Carolina, 2010–2014, accessed September 7, 2015, http://writingcenter.unc.edu/handouts/procrastination/.

6. Robert Burns, "To a Mouse," cited at Poetry Foundation, accessed November 25, 2015, http://www.poetryfoundation.org/poem/173072.

WEEK FOUR: TRAINING IN RESOURCEFULNESS

SCRIPTURE MEMORY VERSE
Be diligent in these matters; give yourself wholly to them, so that everyone may see your progress. 1 Timothy 4:15

One social movement that has been growing in popularity lately is buying nothing new. Families make an agreement for a certain length of time not to purchase new things other than food, car repair items, underclothing, medicine, household cleaning supplies, and things needed for home repair. Families report saving on monthly budgets and paying off debt, but more importantly, they become more creative in problem solving and using the resources they have. They shop at thrift stores, make gifts, share objects such as lawn equipment, and trade with friends and neighbors.[1] They learn how to do more with what they have.

Resourcefulness is a wonderful quality. If you are resourceful, you can creatively solve problems. When new situations arise, you are not fazed by the details. You use your imagination to make something new and useful out of something old and worn out. And you use initiative to serve others with the problems they face. Resourcefulness is certainly a trait of those who take on leadership.

Jesus demonstrated resourcefulness. He turned water into wine, took a few fish and some bread and fed thousands, and walked on water to reach His disciples. Because He was God-on-Earth, He could perform many miracles—tasks we could never accomplish. However, He was also resourceful in human ways—in the ways He drew on earthly resources, adapted to situations, used time well, and asked for what He needed. This week, you will again walk with Christ as He lived out His life resourcefully.

—— DAY 1: LEARN FROM HISTORY
Lord, in school my teachers said we study history to learn from it and not repeat its mistakes. Give me discernment so I will grow in Your wisdom daily. In Jesus's name, amen.

Resourceful people learn from past history. They know mistakes can be costly—wasting time, resources, and energy. So, when faced with the possibility of repeating the mistake, they take a different course. Jesus had three short years in ministry. We know He had a sense of His life's timeline because right at the beginning of His ministry, He told His mother, "My time has not yet come" (John 2:4). The right timing is everything for a resourceful person. Read Matthew 12:9-21. Why did the Pharisees ask Jesus if it was lawful to heal on the Sabbath (see verse 10)?

_____

_____

_____

Nonetheless, how did Jesus help the man with the shriveled hand (see verse 13)?

_____

_____

_____

How did the legalistic Pharisees respond to this healing (see verse 14)?

_____

_____

_____

Why did Jesus withdraw from that place (see verse 15)?

_____

_____

_____

The crowds continued to follow Jesus for His healing touch. What did He warn them not to do (see verse 16)?

_____

_____

_____

Jesus was the prophesied Messiah. Fill in the blanks from verses 18-21:
He will proclaim —————— to the nations. He will not —————— or cry out; no one will —————— his voice in the streets. A bruised reed he will not ——————, and a smoldering wick he will not —————— out, till he —————— justice to ——————. In his name the nations will put their ——————.

Jesus knew He had to be careful not to perform miracles in venues that His opposition would observe. He needed time to mentor His disciples and teach the masses before it was His time to head to the cross. He saw the Pharisees were out to get Him, so there were times He avoided them so His time on earth would not be cut short. As you think about your health-related past, what is one mistake from which you can learn? How could this help develop your resourcefulness?

_____

_____

_____

Lord, I have not always made good choices, but I can learn from my mistakes. Remind me when I am headed in that same direction so I live a healthier life. In Jesus's name, amen.

—— DAY 2: BE FLEXIBLE

Father, I might have a certain mindset at times that might not dovetail with Your plan. Show me how to be flexible so I am walking in sync with You. In Jesus's name, amen.

Stanford University psychologist Carol Dweck recently turned some ideas upside down when she wrote about why brains and talent don't guarantee success—and why they could even stymie it.[2] She also said that praise can actually jeopardize success and productivity.

Dweck states, "In a fixed mindset, people believe their basic qualities, like their intelligence or talent, are simply fixed traits . . . In a growth mindset, people believe that their most basic abilities can be developed through dedication and hard work—brains and talent are just the starting point. This view creates a love of learning and a resilience that is essential for great accomplishment. Virtually all great people have had these qualities."[3]

All of this makes sense in light of what we find in the life of Christ. He took traditional teachings and rules about behavior and interpreted them differently than they had been. This is seen in the incident in which spies—scribes, teachers of the law—tried to trip Him up so He could be handed over to the authority of Roman officials. Read Luke 20:20-26. What was the spies' question (see verse 22)?

_____

_____

What do you think the spies expected Jesus would say?

_____

_____

_____

What did Jesus know (see verse 23)? What two requests did He then make (see verse 24)?

_____

_____

_____

How did the spies respond to Jesus's question about the portrait and inscription (verse 24)?

_____

_____

_____

What was Jesus's answer (see verse 25)?

_____

_____

_____

The spies' question was a setup. If Jesus agreed to pay the taxes, He would seem to be a pawn of the governing Romans. However, if He advised against paying taxes, the spies could have reported Him to Caesar as being a dissident. How was Jesus's response an example of a flexible mindset? How did He use the government's own coin to illustrate His answer?

_____

_____

_____

We often limit our thinking to our own experience and underrated view of ourselves. In doing so, we may conform our minds to patterns that have not been healthy or beneficial. In Romans 12:2, Paul says, "Do not conform to the pattern of this world, but be transformed by the renewing of your mind." Our Creator has made us in His likeness, and He has given each of us creative gifts. We need to read His Word and ask Him to help us see creative solutions so as to be more flexibly resourceful. Write a prayer asking God to give you a creative solution to a concern that you have. Then look in the days ahead for His answer.

_____

_____

_____

Lord, thank You that Your Word can renew my mind and give me creative ways at looking at the challenges of my life. In Jesus's name, amen.

—— DAY 3: DELEGATE

Father, show me how to draw on the strength and assistance of others so I do not become weary in trying to do everything myself. In Jesus's name, amen.

Have you ever wondered why Jesus's time on earth was so short? Why didn't He stay longer? Perhaps He cut His ministry short because He knew that more people could come to the faith through the disciples and other believers. Even when He was alive, Jesus delegated responsibility so as to expand the influence of His ministry. Read Luke 9:1-6. Before Jesus sent out His twelve disciples (Simon, whom He named Peter; his brother Andrew; brothers James and John; Philip; Bartholomew, also called Nathanael; Matthew, also called Levi; Thomas, also called Didymus; James, the son of Alphaeus; Simon the Zealot, Judas, the son of James; and Judas Iscariot), He equipped them in three different ways. What were those ways (see verse 1)?

_____

_____

_____

What tasks did He give them to accomplish (see verse 2)?

_____

_____

_____

As we delegate tasks to others at home, at work, or in a ministry or volunteer position, we can learn from Jesus's example of how He provides instruction to the disciples. What are some of His mandates for their journey (see verses 3-5)?

_____

_____

_____

What are the results of the disciples' travels (see verse 6)?

_____

_____

_____

Jesus's delegation allowed more ground to be covered. More importantly, the disciples experienced God's power working through them as people were healed "everywhere" (Luke 9:6). They are no longer mere bystanders but vehicles of God's power. Likewise, as we learn to delegate some of our responsibilities, we empower others to learn new skills, develop latent talents, and exercise God-given giftings. Children begin to take an investment in their family when they are given responsibilities at home. Ministry helpers become leaders when given the chance to serve in greater capacities. Employees develop management skills when they are allowed to teach and supervise others. Delegating tasks is a win-win strategy for all concerned! Think of at least one task you could delegate to someone else that would lighten your load. Write it down here and then pray about approaching that person.

_____

_____

_____

Father God, show me how to manage the many tasks in my life, because I sincerely want to live as an efficient steward of the time You have given me. In Jesus's name, amen.

—— DAY 4: ASK FOR HELP

Father, I recognize that others may not notice when I need help, so embolden me to honestly share my needs when I am stretched thin. In Jesus's name, amen.

A common expression we often hear is, "Let me know if I can help." But how many times do we follow through and make a request of that person when we are in need? Perhaps we feel awkward about asking—thinking the timing is inconvenient or that what the person had in mind is too much to handle. Often we simply do not want to be rejected, so we do not ask at all. And so we suffer in silence, not taking advantage of a willing helper and depriving that person of the opportunity to bless us. Think of a time when someone helped you—bringing over a meal or helping you with your car or running an errand. How did that make you feel? How do you think the other person felt?

_____

_____

_____

One of the ways Jesus demonstrated resourcefulness was by allowing others to help with physical needs. Read Mark 14:12-16. What was the need Jesus and His disciples had (see verse 12)?

_____

_____

_____

What did Jesus instruct the two disciples to do to meet the need for a meeting place (see verses 13-15)?

_____

_____

_____

Clearly, Jesus already had asked the owner of the house if He and His disciples could meet in what is now referred to as the Upper Room. While we might only remember the disciples and Jesus partaking bread and wine at this meal, the full Passover meal would have been more elaborate—with the recitation of Scripture over several hours and a meal of unleavened bread, wine, bitter herbs, sauce, and lamb. This Last Supper would have been a festive feast with many preparations, so the request for use of the room was significant. When the two disciples made their connection in Jerusalem (see verse 16), what did they find? And what did they do?

_____

_____

_____

Read Luke 19:1-9. What two-part request did Jesus make of Zacchaeus (see verse 5)?

_____

_____

_____

How does Zacchaeus respond (see verse 6)?

_____

_____

_____

What are three results of Zacchaeus's welcoming Jesus to his home—two that bless others and one that blesses him (see verses 8-9?

_____

_____

_____

Asking people to help taps into the gifts, talents, time, and even financial resources they have. While it may be awkward to make a request of someone, most people are more than willing to do what they can to lend a hand. So, how can you help someone in your First Place for Health group this week? Pray about being a blessing!

Lord, helping others brings me joy. Remind me of that when I need others' help so I am not reticent when someone says, "Just let me know how I can help!" In Jesus's name, amen.

—— DAY 5: USE TIME WISELY

Father, with so many social distractions these days it is easy for me to let time slip through my fingers. Help me weigh my choices as my day is laid out before You. In Jesus' name, amen.

Our hands and our minds are our God-given resources meant to do God-ordained work on this earth. As Eugene Peterson writes, "The Bible begins with the announcement 'In the beginning God created'—not 'sat majestic in the heavens,' not 'was filled with beauty and love.' . . . The week of creation was a week of work. The days are described not by their weather conditions and not by their horoscope readings: Genesis 1 is a journal of work. We live in a universe and in a history where God is working. Before anything else, work is an activity of God. . . . We have models of creation, acts of redemption, examples of help and compassion, paradigms of comfort and salvation. One of the reasons that Christians read Scripture repeatedly is to find out just how God works in Jesus Christ so that we can work in the name of Jesus Christ."[4]

Time is a precious commodity, a gift from God. Christ clearly saw every encounter as an opportunity to speak His Father's truth, to explain eternity in understandable images, and to give the opportunity for people to make a decision to follow Him. Every moment, we have the opportunity to be God's instrument wherever we are—at home, in the workplace . . . even in the drive-through at a Starbucks when we need a quick drink.

One day, Jesus was taking a shortcut through Samaria to get from Judea in the south to Galilee in the north. He was tired and rested by a well at about noon. He needed a drink, but He didn't have the means for getting one out of the well. So, when a Samaritan woman came along, He asked if she would give Him a drink. Read the story in John 4:1-30. How did Jesus turn the conversation into a spiritual discussion (see verses 9-10)?

_____

_____

_____

How did Jesus get the woman to understand He was no ordinary passerby (see verses 16-20)?

_____

_____

_____

What did Jesus say would help the woman know that He was the One who could explain everything to her (see verses 25-26)?

_____

_____

_____

Jesus was merely seeking a drink, but His conversation turned into an opportunity to speak truth. Because of that simple meeting, the woman went back to her town (she even left her water jar at the well!) and said, "Come, see a man who told me everything I ever did. Could this be the Messiah?" (John 4:29). So the whole town went to the well to check out the stranger who claimed to be the Messiah. For Jesus every chance meeting was another opportunity to point people to His Father and introduce

Himself as God's Son. As you think through how you typically spend a weekday, list a few ways you could use your time more efficiently for the kingdom.

_____

_____

_____

Lord, thank You for how You ordered the universe, with the sunrise and sunset and the seasons of change. May You be pleased with how I use the days You have given me. In Jesus's name, amen.

—— DAY 6: REFLECTION AND APPLICATION

Father, Your Word is one of the greatest tools from which I can clarify direction, discern truth from lies, and draw strength. Keep me faithful in my study, Lord! In Jesus's name, amen.

One of the greatest resources from which you can draw is the Bible. In fact, it could be called a Problem-Solving Manual because it provides comfort in times of mourning, hope in times of despair, direction in times of confusion, and fortification in times of temptation. Sometimes you might not be certain of how God might view a problem you are facing, or you might feel God has been silent on a particular issue. However, the Bible gives tremendous guidance.

Jesus quoted from the Old Testament dozens of times. When the chief priests and teachers of the law harassed Him after some children praised Him, He quoted from Psalm 8:2 (see Matthew 21:16). He quoted Isaiah 53:12 to His disciples when explaining to them that He must die a sinner's death (Luke 22:37). When He taught during the Sermon on the Mount, He quoted from Exodus 20:13 and 21:12 (see Matthew 5:21-22). Other than His relationship and position with His heavenly Father, the Scripture in Jesus's heart and mind was His greatest resource.

When you take on a new challenge, you might find you are soon facing all kinds of temptation that could cause you to falter. Scripture is a problem-solving resource you can use during those times. Read Matthew 4:1-11. What were the three different ways that Jesus was tempted? How did Jesus respond?

	How Jesus Was Tempted	How He Responded
vv. 3-4		
vv. 5-7		
vv. 8-10		

After Jesus's responses, what did the devil do? What did the angels do (see verse 11)?

_____

_____

_____

_____

The enemy cannot stand in the presence of the truth of God's Word, and you can use it to help you live a victorious life. One way to use Scripture is to personalize it. Fill in the example below—the same Scripture Jesus used when the devil tempted Him (Matthew 4:4, taken from Deuteronomy 8:3)—plugging your name in the blank:

_____ *shall not live on bread alone, but on every word that comes from the mouth of God.*

Meditate on that verse. Store it in your heart. And when you are tempted, draw it out like a sword and slice that temptation into bits!

Lord, thank You for the power of Your Word. May I not take it lightly but feed on it daily so that Your power fills me in times of weakness. In Jesus's name, amen.

—— DAY 7: REFLECTION AND APPLICATION

Father, it is easy to let time slip through my fingers with so many social distractions these days. Help me weigh my choices as my day is laid out before You. In Jesus's name, amen.

In Paul's first letter to the younger Timothy, he wrote, "Train yourself to be godly. For physical training is of some value, but godliness has value for all things, holding promise for both the present life and the life to come" (1 Timothy 4:7-8). The word *train* in verse 7 is more strongly translated *discipline* in the *NASB* and *exercise* in the *KJV*. The word comes from the Greek *gumnazo*, which was used with physical training, such as gymnastics, but also with the training of the mind. Paul clearly wanted Timothy to work vigorously at his training in godliness so that he will be a testimony to others.

When we have had a godly workout—studying God's Word, praying faithfully, memorizing Scripture—we ourselves are a resource that God can use. We will be trained and strengthened for the race set before us. Paul continued his encouragement to Timothy by stating, "Set an example for the believers in speech, in life, in love, in faith and in purity. Until I come, devote yourself to the public reading of Scripture, to preaching and to teaching. Do not neglect your gift" (1 Timothy 4:12-14).

The inspiration for our spiritual workout, Paul said, is "the living God, who is the Savior of all people" (verse 10). When we exercise discipline to develop godly characteristics such as resourcefulness, God empowers us to exercise our gifts in such a way that we become examples to those newer in the faith.

Reread 1 Timothy 4:15, your memory verse for the week. What will be the effect of your efforts to become more Christ-like?

_____

_____

_____

Whom do you hope to influence with your faith? Write the names below and share at least one name with your First Place 4 Health friends for the purpose of prayer.

_____

_____

_____

Lord, thank You for sending Your Son, Jesus, to provide an example of how I might live more resourcefully. May my life stand out in such a way that others are drawn to You. In Jesus's name, amen.

Notes

1. Jen Hansard, "The Compact: Not Buy Anything New for a Year," Family Sponge, December 12, 2012, accessed September 8, 2015, http://familysponge.com/parenting/inspired-parenting/the-compact-not-buy-anything-new-for-a-year/.

2. Carol Dweck, Mindset: The New Psychology of Success (New York: Ballantine Books, 2007).

3. Carol Dweck, "What Is Mindset," Mindset.com, accessed September 9, 2015, http://mindsetonline.com/.

4. Eugene H. Peterson, A Long Obedience in the Same Direction (Downers Grove, IL: InterVarsity Press, 2000), 108-109.

WEEK FIVE: TRAINING IN WISDOM

SCRIPTURE MEMORY VERSE
The fear of the LORD is the beginning of wisdom; all who follow his precepts have good understanding. To him belongs eternal praise. Psalm 111:10

In the fall of Jesus's third and final year of ministry, His own brothers encouraged Him to go to Judea during the Feast of the Tabernacles to do miracles publicly. John tells us Jesus's "own brothers did not believe in him" (John 7:5), so He may have been an embarrassment or an annoyance to them (see Matthew 13:55-57). Sometime after His brothers left for the feast, which was a weeklong celebration of the harvest, He went as well.

About halfway through the feast, Jesus went to the Temple courts and began to teach. John stated, "The Jews there were amazed and asked, 'How did this man get such learning without having been taught?' Jesus answered, 'My teaching is not my own. It comes from the one who sent me. If anyone chooses to do the will of God will find out whether my teaching comes from God or whether I speak on my own. Whoever who speaks on their own does so to gain personal glory, but he who seeks the glory of the one who sent him is a man of truth; there is nothing false about him. Has not Moses given you the law? Yet not one of you keeps the law. Why are you trying to kill me?'" (John 7:15-19).

Jesus's wisdom continues to amaze people even today. His teachings and His responses to His questioners demonstrated sophisticated scholarship, intelligence, clear judgment, and circumspection—delivered in language and with examples that even common people could understand. That kind of wisdom is worth pursuing every day and for a lifetime. This week, you will learn about practical ways to become a person of wisdom.

—— DAY 1: SEEK MENTORS
Father, I have much to learn. I pray that I can glean from the wisdom of others and apply their teachings to my life. In Jesus's name, amen.

The only story we have about Jesus's childhood is that of His being found after going missing for three days—when he was only 12 years old. Review the story in Luke 2:41-52. Where did Joseph and Mary find Jesus? Who was with Him (see verse 46)?

_____
_____
_____

What two things was Jesus doing (see verse 46)?

_____
_____
_____

How did people who heard the boy Jesus respond to Him (see verse 47)?

_____
_____
_____

Jesus, a young adolescent, had been missing from His parents for three days. How did they respond when they found Him (see verse 48)? What did they say to Him?

_____
_____
_____

What was Jesus's response to His mother's question (see verse 49)?

_____
_____
_____

We know from Luke 1:30-38 that Mary knew her child, Jesus, would be the Messiah, the Son of the Most High God. Certainly, she must have had some conflicting emotions on seeing Him listening and speaking with teachers in the Temple. What does Scripture say were Mary's initial reaction, second response, and her later response (see Luke 2:48, 50-51)?

_____
_____
_____

Luke 2:52 tells us that Jesus grew in wisdom, in stature, and in favor with God and man. What do each of those ways of growth mean?

Wisdom:

_____
_____
_____

Stature:

_____
_____
_____

Favor with God:

_____
_____
_____

Favor with man:

_____
_____
_____

Just as Jesus sought the wisdom of others, you can too. In the space below, list the names of people whose teaching and advice you trust—people from whom you could learn. These names could include authors whose writing spurs you on to growth.

_____
_____
_____

If you are young in the faith, consider asking someone to mentor you. If you are mature in the faith, perhaps you could mentor someone younger. Give some thought and prayer to this idea.

Lord, I trust that You will continue to provide teachers or mentor figures in my life who will encourage me to study Your Word and apply it to my life. In Jesus's name, amen.

—— DAY 2: PAY ATTENTION

Father, I want to gain greater understanding when You are speaking to me through Your Word, through prayer, through others, or through the circumstances in my life. In Jesus's name, amen.

In *Experiencing God*, Henry Blackaby and Claude King write, "God speaks by the Holy Spirit through the Bible, prayer, circumstances, and the church to reveal Himself, His purposes, and His ways."[1] Sometimes, however, you may get caught up in your own tasks instead of paying attention to how God is communicating with you. Blackaby and King explain, "If you were to record a whole day in your life you might find that your prayers, your attitudes, your thoughts, everything about that day is radically self-centered. You may not be seeing things from God's perspective. . . . When He becomes the Lord of your life, He alone has the right to be . . . the Focus in your life, the Initiator in your life, the Director of your life."[2] Read John 10:25-28. Jesus called His followers "sheep." What two things does He say His sheep do (see verse 27)?

_____

_____

What are the benefits of listening to Jesus and following Him (see verses 27-28)?

_____

_____

_____

Read Mark 9:2-7. Jesus had taken Peter, James, and John with Him up a mountain, where two amazing events happened. First, Jesus's clothes were transfigured into a dazzling white. Then visions of Elijah and Moses appeared—and the two men talked with Jesus. Peter then made a suggestion to construct three shelters—for Jesus, Moses, and Elijah. What does the Father say at this point from the cloud (see verse 7)?

_____

_____

_____

Why would God need to tell Jesus's disciples to pay attention?

_____

_____

What can be gained by being quiet and listening?

_____
_____
_____

What wisdom could be gained by paying attention through these means?

The Bible:

_____
_____
_____

Prayer:

_____
_____
_____

Other people:

_____
_____
_____

Circumstances:

_____
_____
_____

Lord, thank You for providing ways for me to gain wisdom. I will pay attention as You direct me through Your Word, prayer, other people, and circumstances. In Jesus's name, amen.

—— DAY 3: WEIGH DECISIONS

Father, You have given me a mind to develop and use for good. Guide me to weigh ideas against Scripture and make decisions with godly confidence. In Jesus's name, amen.

What do you do when you have to make a critical decision? Some people make pros-and-cons lists, some people do research, and some go with their gut instinct.

These differences may have to do with personality. Some people are meticulous and carefully plan their next steps. Others are carefree and make decisions based on experience and feelings. In the Gospels we see a *deliberate* Jesus. Before beginning His ministry, He fasted in the desert for forty days (see Luke 4:1-2). Before He chose His disciples, He spent the night praying (see 6:12). Before He allowed Himself to be arrested and hung on the cross, He spent a significant chunk of a night praying in Gethsemane (see 22:39-46). What do you think prayer has to do with decision-making?

_____

_____

_____

Recall a time when you prayed before making an important decision. What effect did prayer have on the outcome?

_____

_____

_____

Remember a time when you made a wrong decision. What could have helped you make the right decision?

_____

_____

_____

In contrast to Jesus's deliberate approach to decision-making, His disciples made decisions to follow Him on the spot. When Jesus called the fisherman brothers Simon Peter and Andrew to follow Him, the two men left their nets and joined him at once (see Matthew 4:18-20). A bit later when Jesus called two other fishermen brothers, James and John, to follow Him, they left their boat and their father, Zebedee, immediately (see verses 21-22). Luke reports the other eight disciples were chosen that same day (see Luke 6:13-16), so they likely did not hestitate either. Do you sense a commonality in these examples? Explain.

_____

_____

_____

So, what is the best method for decision-making? Should you research, study, and pray before making decisions? Or should you just go with what seems right in the moment? There is actually no conflict in teaching here. Jesus had to confer with God during those turning-point times in His ministry. The disciples were doing the same, except they were speaking face-to-face with God the Son. The one thread in the disciples' decisions to leave their work and families immediately and follow Jesus was the Savior Himself. He was doing the calling—speaking to their hearts, minds, and souls—and hearing His voice beckon was all they needed to know. You, too, can be spontaneous in your decision-making when God is calling to your heart, mind, and soul. Have you ever sensed God's clear nudging as you faced a decision? If so, explain the circumstances and how you knew God was clearly speaking direction into your life.

_____

_____

_____

Lord, make my mind, heart, and soul in tune with Yours, so I can clearly sense Your will as I face the important decisions in my life. In Jesus's name, amen.

—— DAY 4: LEARN FROM MISTAKES

Father, thank You that Your mercy and grace cover over any mistakes that I make. Let me learn from them so I represent you well. In Jesus's name, amen.

Sometimes we think our mistakes disqualify us. If that were so, why would Jesus have told Peter that He would build His church on him (see Mathew 16:18)? After all, Peter said some ridiculous things and made significant mistakes. Perhaps Jesus knew he would learn from his mistakes and live up to his name, Peter, which means "rock." One of the first times we read of Peter in action is when he saw Jesus walk on the surface of the Sea of Galilee. Read Matthew 14:22-33. What mistake did Peter make (see verse 30)?

_____

_____

_____

How did Jesus respond to Peter (see verse 31)?

_____

_____

WEEK FIVE TRAINING IN WISDOM

Another instance that calls Peter's leadership ability into question occurred shortly after Jesus had been teaching in villages near Caesarea Philippi. Read Mark 8:27-33. What proclamation about Jesus did Peter make (see verse 29)?

_____

_____

_____

When Jesus later told His disciples that He must suffer, be rejected by authorities, and be killed, followed by resurrection, how did Peter respond in front of the other disciples (see verse 32)?

_____

_____

_____

Again, how did Jesus respond to Peter (see verse 33)?

_____

_____

_____

Just after Jesus was arrested, Peter did something impetuous. Read John 18:10-11. What did Peter do (see verse 10)?

_____

_____

_____

How did Jesus respond to Peter (see verse 11)?

_____

_____

_____

When Jesus and the disciples were having the Last Supper together, Peter claimed he would follow Jesus to prison and death (see Luke 22:33). Jesus told Peter, "Before the rooster crows today, you will deny three times that you know me" (verse 34). Read John 18:15-18, 25-27. To what three people does Peter, in fact, deny knowing Jesus (see verses 16-17, 25-27)?

_____

_____

_____

Clearly, Jesus had quite a time mentoring Peter! The disciple walked on water but then sank from lack of faith (see Matthew 14:22-31). He contradicted Jesus in front of the other disciples and was reprimanded (see Mark 8:32-33). He chopped off the ear of the high priest's servant and again was scolded publicly (see John 18:10-11). He then denied Christ three times (see Luke 22:55-62).

Yet after Jesus's resurrection, when Christ appeared to the disciples, He restored Peter and called him to leadership (see John 21:15-23). Despite having doubts, despite impetuous words and mistakes, Peter learned from his history and from Christ's confidence in him. A man who said and did the wrong things—seemingly over and over—became the bold proclaimer of the gospel message and helped create a movement that became the Christian church.

People are bound to make mistakes, but they can change by deciding to get healthier and become more Christ-like. How have you learned from your mistakes? Perhaps you would like to share a story with your First Place for Health group to encourage them.

Lord, I am grateful that You overlook the mistakes of Your people and use them anyway. Help me to learn from my mistakes and become an effective witness for You. In Jesus's name, amen.

—— DAY 5: DISCERN TRUTH

Father, as I am bombarded by the noise of the world, help me discern Your truth. Show me how to weigh others' words and actions against the truth of Your Word. In Jesus's name, amen.

People say actions speak louder than words. This is a message Jesus also proclaimed when others were trying to figure out if He was the prophesied Messiah. Read Matthew 11:1-19. The man known as John the Baptist was actually a relative of Jesus (see Luke 1:5-45). John was called the last prophet of the Old Covenant, and his purpose was to prepare the way for the coming Messiah—Jesus. From prison, John heard about Christ's miracles and healings. What question did John send to Jesus through his messengers (see Matthew 11:3)?

_____

_____

_____

How did Jesus respond (see verses 4-6)?

_____

_____

_____

Jesus then spoke to the crowd about John and his ministry—effectively explaining what the prophet's purpose was. Jesus said that John was meant as a messenger to prepare people for the coming of the Christ. Jesus concluded this speech by saying, "But wisdom is proved right by her deeds" (verse 19). What did He mean by this?

_____

_____

_____

Jesus did prove that He was the Christ, the long-expected Messiah who brought salvation to all who would believe. He performed miracles, interpreted Scripture in ways that had never before communicated such graceful wisdom, and, in a final redemptive act, went to the cross to atone for the sins of those who choose to believe He is the Son of God. His actions proved the truth of His words. Similarly, as you follow your Personal Trainer in developing Christ-like characteristics, actual follow-through will be important as you make new commitments. How could your actions speak more loudly than words in your own life?

_____

_____

_____

Lord, may I be a person of wisdom, living a life of integrity not only by saying the right thing but also by doing the right thing. In Jesus's name, amen.

—— DAY 6: REFLECTION AND APPLICATION

Father, keep me childlike in my faith—but hungry for learning more about You each day. In Jesus's name, amen.

Toward the end of one teaching session, Jesus said, "I praise you, Father, Lord of heaven and earth, because you have hidden these things from the wise and learned, and revealed them to little children. Yes, Father, for this is what you were pleased to do" (Matthew 11:25-26). Jesus had been observing that the "wise and learned" were anything but. Certainly, the leaders had studied the law of the Old Testament and were well-versed in what it said, but they did not recognize that He was the embodied fulfillment of it.

In contrast, one refreshing quality of children is their insatiable desire to learn. They listen to their teachers and trust them. Children do not question the educational background or integrity of those teaching them. They believe (and even love) their teachers, take their studies seriously, and grow in leaps and bounds. Being a willing learner—not a know-it-all—is important to our growing in wisdom.

The Bible was meant to document God's love for us and His pursuit of a relationship with us. By studying the patriarchs, the judges, the kings, the prophets, and the wisdom writings, we can see God's loving guidance and frequent correction of a people who were determined to mess up more often than not. Then God did the craziest thing: He came to earth in the form of Jesus Christ, fulfilling Old Testament prophecies of a Messiah who would become the final piece of understanding so all would know the love of God for the sake of eternity. The Bible is the story of God's sacred romance of all humankind—His quest to rescue us from our mixed up selves and sweep us unto Himself. The Bible can breathe life into us.

As an 18-year-old college freshman, my now-husband Craig found this to be true when he attended the University of California, Berkeley, during the Vietnam War protest period. In those day, young people were questioning every tradition, including the faith. One day as Craig sat in Sproul Plaza, the center of anti-war protests, he met a Christian campus ministry worker named Neil who asked if he believed Christ was the Son of God. Although Craig had been raised in the church, he was not sure what he believed about Christ. Neil challenged him to read the Bible to discover the truth for himself . . . so Craig did. He started in the book of Genesis and read all the way through to Revelation. "It made sense," he says, "so I believed."

Reading the Bible daily can infuse the life-giving truth of God's Word into your veins. How could faithful study of the Bible develop wisdom that would spur your growth in the following core areas of First Place for Health?

Physical

_____
_____
_____

Mental

_____
_____
_____

Emotional

_____
_____
_____

Spiritual

_____
_____
_____

Lord, Your Word is a lamp that illuminates wisdom. May I not neglect my studies so that I may learn more about You each day and become more like Christ. In Jesus's name, amen.

—— DAY 7: REFLECTION AND APPLICATION

Father, keep me childlike in my faith—but hungry for learning more about You each day. In Jesus's name, amen.

Fill in the blanks for Psalm 111:10, this week's memory verse:

The _____ of the _____ is the beginning of_____;
all who _____ his_____ have good_____. To him
belongs _____ _____.

According to this passage, where does wisdom start for believers?

_____

_____

_____

In this context the word *fear* means "reverential awe." When we revere someone, we respect that person and give great honor to him or her. Awe is an emotion that combines dread, veneration (a form of *revere*), and wonder, inspired by authority or the sacred. As believers our wisdom can begin when we give God all the honor and praise and glory that we possibly can. He is the Creator of the universe and has fashioned all creatures, including humans with skin, bones, heart, brains, and soul. Not acknowledging the Giver of Life is either ignorance or arrogance, because apart from God we can only generate widsom incompletely.

Notice from the memory verse that the fear of the Lord is the *beginning* of wisdom. This is the best starting place. In *Your God Is Too Safe*, Mark Buchanan writes it is a "fearful thing to fall into the hands of the living God. He's dangerous, not safe at all. And yet there is something far more fearful and dangerous than to fall into His hands: to *not* fall into His hands."[3]

Buchanan reminds readers of C.S. Lewis's classic chronicle *The Lion, The Witch and the Wardrobe*. He notes that in the story, "The children—Peter, Susan, Lucy, and Edmund—enter Narnia through a wardrobe in their uncle's home. Edmund has already given allegiance to the witch and sneaks off to join ranks with her. The other three children go to the home of the Beavers, a wary but hospitable pair. Mr. and Mrs. Beaver tell the children that they will take them to see the King, Aslan."[4] The children then asked more about Aslan:

> "Is—is he a man?" asked Lucy.
> "Aslan a man!" said Mr. Beaver sternly. "Certainly not. I tell you he is the King of the wood and the son of the great Emperor-beyond-the-Sea. Don't you know who is the King of Beasts? Aslan is a lion–*the* Lion, the great Lion."
> "Ooh," said Susan, "I'd thought he was a man. Is he—quite safe? I shall feel rather nervous about meeting a lion."
> "That you will, dearie, and no mistake," said Mrs. Beaver; "if there's anyone who can appear before Aslan without their knees knocking, they're either braver than most or else just silly."

"Then he isn't safe?" said Lucy.

"Safe?" said Mr. Beaver; "don't you hear what Mrs. Beaver tells you? Who said anything about safe? 'Course he isn't safe. But he's good. He's the king, I tell you."

"I'm longing to see him," said Peter, "even if I do feel frightened when it comes to the point."[5]

The point is that God can nurture and build wisdom in us when we acknowledge that He is Lord and we are the work of His hands. That means we are still in process—we do not have all the keys to understanding—so reading His Word, following His nudgings, and serving Him in reverential awe will get us on our own Narnia paths.

Lord, You are good and worthy of all my honor and praise. Your Word gives understanding to my heart and helps me see how You want to protect me from slipping into my own mistaken directions and heartache. Like Peter, I long for Your presence. In Jesus's name, amen.

Notes

1. Henry T. Blackaby and Claude V. King, *Experiencing God* (Nashville, TN: LifeWay Press, 1990), 225.

2. Blackaby and King, *Experiencing God*, 99.

3. Mark Buchanan, *Your God Is Too Safe* (Sisters, OR: Multnomah, 2001), 30.

4. Buchanan, *Your God*, 31.

5. C.S. Lewis, *The Lion, the Witch and the Wardrobe* (New York: HarperCollins, 1978), 86.

WEEK SIX: TRAINING IN FAITHFULNESS

SCRIPTURE MEMORY VERSE

His master replied, "Well done, good and faithful servant! You have been faithful with a few things; I will put you in charge of many things. Come and share in your master's happiness!" Matthew 25:23

Jesus exemplified the characteristic of faithfulness. After the resurrection, He appeared to the disciples and lived among them for 40 days, giving them "many convincing proofs" and speaking about the kingdom of God (Acts 1:3). In Acts 1:4-5, Luke reported, "On one occasion, while he was eating with them, he gave them this command: 'Do not leave Jerusalem, but wait for the gift my Father promised, which you have heard me speak about. For John baptized with water, but in a few days you will be baptized with the Holy Spirit.'"

Jesus then told them they would receive power when the Holy Spirit came on them, and they would be His "witnesses in Jerusalem, and in all Judea and Samaria, and to the ends of the earth" (verse 8). Ten days later, on the Day of Pentecost, a "sound like the blowing of a violent wind came from heaven and filled the whole house" where the disciples were staying (2:2). Just as Jesus had promised, the Holy Spirit fell on the believers.

Peter, empowered by the Holy Spirit, spoke to crowd, and they asked what they should do in response to the wonders they were witnessing. Peter replied, "Repent and be baptized, every one of you, in the name of Jesus Christ for the forgiveness of your sins. And you will receive the gift of the Holy Spirit. The promise is for you and your children and for all who are far off—for all whom the Lord our God will call" (verses 38-39).

About 3,000 people committed themselves to following Christ that day (see verse 41). Just as the Father was faithful to send the Messiah and raise Christ from the dead after three days, He was also faithful to fulfill Jesus's promise and send the Holy Spirit. Jesus promised He would never leave us (see Matthew 28:20), and it is His faithfulness to His family, His friends, His work on earth, and His Father that inspire us to be faithful as well.

—— DAY 1: BE FAITHFUL TO FAMILY

Father, thank You for giving me my family. While none of us is perfect, I am grateful for daily opportunities to live out Your love with them. In Jesus's name, amen.

One of the most touching scenes in Scripture is when Jesus speaks from the cross to His disciple John, who several times in his Gospel refers to himself as "the disciple whom he loved." Read John 19:25-27. Who is standing near the cross (see verses 25-26)?

_____

_____

_____

What does Jesus tell His mother (see verse 26)?

_____

_____

_____

What does Jesus tell John (see verse 27)?

_____

_____

_____

What do you think was Jesus implying by these remarks?

_____

_____

_____

Given that Jesus had several brothers, His statements might seem odd. After all, the brothers could look after their mother, Mary, couldn't they? However, in John 7:5 we learn that "even his own brothers did not believe in him," and because Jesus's brothers were apparently not at the crucifixion, He might have been concerned about His mother's welfare after His death. After all, Mary had believed in Him—potentially isolating herself from the unfaithful brothers.

John is the one disciple with Jesus at the foot of the cross. Because John is faithful, Jesus entrusts him with His mother's future care. That's what families do: protect, defend, care for, and honor one another . . . at least in theory. Even Jesus's family had its struggles. In Luke 8:19-21, we read how Jesus's mother, Mary, and His brothers went to see Him when He was speaking to a crowd. When someone told Jesus they were there, He responded, "My mother and brothers are those who hear God's word and put it into practice" (verse 21).

While this seems like an odd reply, one commentary notes that the family thought Jesus was out of His mind, and they probably wanted to take Him away.[1] Nonetheless, despite any family baggage of the past, Jesus had His mother on His heart just before His death. She was important to Him—and His spoken last-will-and-testament gift was His provision of care through His closest earthly friend, John.

How has family helped you during tough times?

_____
_____
_____

Even if your family has been less than perfect, you can take comfort in knowing that, like Christ, you have a Christian family—"those who hear God's word and put it into practice" (Luke 8:21). How could you demonstrate faithfulness to your family—either your literal family or your Christian family?

_____
_____
_____

Jesus, I love that You demonstrated Your love for Your mother at the end of Your life on earth. Show me how I also can think of others' needs in my family. In Jesus's name, amen.

—— DAY 2: BE FAITHFUL TO FRIENDS

Father, thank You for the friendships in my life. Please develop faithfulness in me so I can be Your hands and feet—and love on them as You would. In Jesus's name, amen.

Jesus was faithful to those who extended friendship to Him. So He was heartbroken when He learned that His friend Lazarus had died. Read John 11:1-44. Why did Jesus delay traveling to Lazarus's side when He learned he was sick (see verse 4)?

_____

_____

_____

Why didn't the disciples want Him to travel to help Lazarus (see verse 8)?

_____

_____

_____

Jesus apparently knew that Lazarus was dead when He left two days later. When He arrived in Bethany at the home of Martha and Mary, Lazarus's sisters, what was Martha's two-part response (see verses 21-22)?

_____

_____

_____

Jesus delayed His arrival so God would be glorified through Him when He raised Lazarus from the dead. The Lord of Life knew that His friend would breathe life on earth once more. Even so, what was Jesus's reaction when He saw Mary and others weeping at the tomb? What was His reaction when He saw His friend Lazarus lying dead? (See verses 33-35.)

_____

_____

_____

The story ends happily: Jesus raised Lazarus from the dead, and people came to faith in the Lord of Life. However, Jesus still wept when He saw others heartbroken and Lazarus lifeless. What does the fact "Jesus wept" (verse 35) tell us about His love and faithfulness for His friends?

_____

_____

_____

What are some practical ways you could demonstrate faithfulness to your friends this week?

_____

_____

_____

Lord, You breathed life back into Lazarus. Show me how I could encourage a friend who needs a little breath of life this week. In Jesus's name, amen.

—— DAY 3: BE FAITHFUL AT WORK

Father, my witness is on the line when I work—both at home and beyond. May I be a person of commitment and integrity as I work in Your name. In Jesus's name, amen.

Faithful workers stick to their commitments, demonstrate focus, and work to please the Lord. As Christians we want our walk to match our talk. James 1:22 says, "Do not merely listen to the word, and so deceive yourselves. Do what it says."

The hard part for us is that once we commit our lives to Christ, others identify us with principles for living laid out across some 2,000 pages of the Bible. Conversely, those who do not believe in Christ are not necessarily accountable to any sort of standards other than ones they create for themselves. We have a nearly impossible level of accountability—and because we are human, we will make mistakes. While we know we are forgiven in a heavenly sense, our errors can create problems for others and can reflect poorly on the Lord we serve.

Read the parable of the shrewd manager in Luke 16:1-15. What had the rich man heard about his manager (see verse 1)? What did the rich man request of the man (see verse 2)?

_____

_____

_____

When the manager learned he had lost his job, what actions did he take to gain favor with the rich man's creditors (see verses 3-7)?

_____

_____

_____

The manager is called *shrewd* because he discounted the debts owed by his master's creditors. In doing so, his master received less than what he was owed, while the manager made points with the creditors. This was a strategy that could help him down the road when he himself was in need. How do you feel about what the manager did? Were these acts of integrity?

_____

_____

_____

Jesus continued by saying the master commended the dishonest manager because of his shrewdness. Jesus then taught that worldly wealth should be used to "gain friends for yourselves, so that when it is gone, you will be welcomed into eternal dwellings" (Luke 16:9). We can invest our money in others, who will then see our care for them and investigate the Christ we serve. What are some ways you could invest in others?

_____

_____

_____

What do we learn about trustworthiness in verses 10-12? Who is trustworthy? Who is not?

_____

_____

_____

In the workplace the employer needs to be able to trust his or her employees. What are some principles a Christian should follow at work—either in the home or in another workplace?

_____

_____

_____

What is a workplace challenge you have had? How could you demonstrate faithful integrity in this regard in the future?

_____

_____

_____

Lord, teach me to be a good example to others as I work. May my witness be clean so that others know I work to serve You and those You love. In Jesus's name, amen.

—— DAY 4: BE FAITHFUL IN MINISTRY

Father, You have given me spiritual giftings that I can use to serve You. I pray that You are honored and pleased with whatever I do for Your sake. In Jesus's name, amen.

The word *talent* has an interesting origin. According to *Merriam-Webster*, a talent was a unit of weight and money in the ancient world. However, the meaning of the word changed because of a parable Jesus told in Matthew 25:14-30. In this story why did the master give differing amounts to the three servants (see verse 15)?

_____

_____

_____

What did each of the men do with the talents they had been given (see verses 16-18)?

_____

_____

_____

How did the master respond to each when he returned (see verses 19-28)?

_____

_____

_____

According to verses 28-30, what will result when we use their talents (God-given gifts and abilities)? How does God feel about those who do not use their talents?

_____

_____

_____

In Romans 12:6-8, Paul lists some of the spiritual gifts God gives to Christ follow-ers: *prophecy, service, teaching, encouragement, giving, leadership,* and *mercy.* He lists additional gifts in 1 Corinthians 12:8-10: *wisdom, knowledge, faith, healing, miracles, discernment (distinguishing between spirits), speaking in unlearned languages, and inter-pretation of those languages.* Others are listed in Ephesians 4:11: *apostleship, evange-*

lism, and *pastoring.* What spiritual gifts do you have? (If you're not sure, ask someone who knows you well.) How have you used your gift, or how could you use it?

_____

_____

_____

Lord, what a privilege it is to serve You in my church, my community, and in the world. Use me to further and build Your kingdom here on earth. In Jesus's name, amen.

—— DAY 5: BE FAITHFUL IN CONFLICT

Father, I am like an ambassador, testifying to You and Your kingdom—such an exciting assignment! Lead me, Lord, as I bear Your witness. In Jesus's name, amen.

It is not difficult to sing God's praises when life is a smooth path with no obstructions. However, our reactions are even more important when people mistreat us. Read Luke 6:27-36 and fill in Jesus's teachings in the following blanks:

_____ your enemies (v. 27).

_____ to those who hate you (v. 27).

_____ those who curse you (v 28).

_____ for those who mistreat you (v. 28).

How might this be opposite from what our natural response might be?

_____

_____

_____

How might others see a reflection of Christ in us if we respond in these gracious and forgiving ways when someone treats us meanly?

_____

_____

_____

You have likely heard the expression, "turn the other cheek." What does this mean? How would you typically respond to someone who criticizes you?

_____

_____

_____

MYplace O FOR BIBLE STUDY

Jesus taught that if someone steals from us, we should give that person something more (see verses 29-30). How do you feel about this?

_____

_____

_____

In verse 31 Jesus gave what would later be called the "Golden Rule" that many people express as one of their core values: "Do to others as you would have them do to you." List at least three examples of how a person could demonstrate the Golden Rule to others.

_____

_____

_____

What is the reasoning Jesus gives for this important principal (see verses 32-36)?

_____

_____

_____

Why should turning the other cheek and treating others as you would want to be treated be a practice for someone who wanted to demonstrate faithfulness to Jesus Christ?

_____

_____

_____

Lord, You blessed those who cursed You and did not lash out at those who crucified You. Help me to be faithful when life is hard and to be faithful to Your example. In Jesus's name, amen.

—— DAY 6: REFLECTION AND APPLICATION

Father, Your faithfulness throughout the generations and the centuries humbles me. You have pursued me and are more than worthy of my faithful love in return. In Jesus's name, amen.

We often hear the word *faithfulness* when speaking about marriage. This is because one of the most important qualities married couples need from each other is faithfulness—the state of being committed to someone regardless of the circumstances.

In the matrimony ceremony, some ministers use the traditional vow for the groom from *The Book of Common Prayer*:

> I, _____, take thee,_____, to my wedded Wife, to have and to hold, from this day forward, for better for worse, for richer for poorer, in sickness and in health, to love and to cherish, till death us do part, according to God's holy ordinance; and thereto I plight thee my troth.[2]

Faithfulness assumes we remain loyal and committed no matter the circumstances. However, even if the marriage has fallen apart, we are still part of an even greater romance—God's pursuit of us. The relationship began with His conversations with Adam and Eve. He continued to pursue His earthly creation through patriarchs such as Abraham, Jacob, and Joseph, and then through the judges.

But with each judge's death, the people again "did evil in the eyes of the LORD" (Judges 3:12). Again and again the people turned away from the God who loved them. Then they called for a king, and God gave them Saul, then David, and then a long succession of many others, as well as prophets who listened for the voice of the Pursuer. However, because the pursued were unfaithful, God's voice eventually faded out for 400 years.

Then the loving God sent His Son, Jesus, so that those who would listen to the call of love would understand *faithfulness* was a person—Jesus Christ. Brent Curtis and John Eldredge call this story of God's pursuit of man the *Sacred Romance*: "We come to know God by coming to know the Sacred Romance he is telling. We come to understand who we are by telling each other our stories in light of the Sacred Romance."[3] All God asks in return is our faithfulness. In Matthew 10:32-33, Jesus teaches, "Whoever acknowledges me before others, I will also acknowledge before my Father in heaven. But whoever disowns me before others, I will disown before my Father in heaven."

In our daily interactions with others, what could be some instances of how we might acknowledge Christ?

_____

_____

_____

Is that a comfortable practice for you? Why or why not?

_____

_____

_____

What does the word *disown* mean to you? How do you think it would feel to be disowned?

_____

_____

_____

How could you demonstrate your faithfulness to God this week?

_____

_____

_____

Lord, thank You for loving me enough to overlook my weaknesses and pursue me. I commit to loving You and promise to acknowledge You before others—with words and with actions that bear out those words. In Jesus's name, amen.

—— DAY 7: REFLECTION AND APPLICATION

Father, one way I can demonstrate my faithfulness is to worship You on the Sabbath. May my faithfulness help preserve Your name throughout the generations. In Jesus's name, amen.

One way to demonstrate our faithfulness to the God we love is to observe His Sabbath—to worship and rest on Sunday. It is sweet irony that setting aside one day each week to worship God and take a restful break provides such refreshment for us as well. Many discussions about the Sabbath relate to wiggle-room analysis of exactly what we need to do to observe this weekly Father's Day. But perhaps a better question is, "What is the Sabbath really about?" Pastor and theologian Tim Keller provides this answer:

> According to the Bible, it is about more than just taking time off. After creating the world, God looked around and saw that "it was very good" (Genesis 1:31). God did not just cease from his labor; he stopped and enjoyed what he had made. What does this mean for us? We need to stop to enjoy God, to enjoy his creation, to

enjoy the fruits of our labor. The whole point of Sabbath is joy in what God has done. . . . In the Bible, Sabbath rest means to cease regularly from and to enjoy the results of your work. It provides balance: "Six days you shall labor and do all your work, but the seventh day is a Sabbath to the Lord your God" (Exodus 20:9–10). Although Sabbath rest receives a much smaller amount of time than work, it is a necessary counterbalance so that the rest of your work can be good and beneficial.[4]

While originally people were not even supposed to prepare a meal on the Sabbath, as that was considered work, Jesus mixed it up in His teachings. We see in Matthew 12:1-14 that He picked grain to eat and healed a man's shriveled hand. Doing good on the Sabbath, Jesus said, was the correct action to take (see Matthew 12:12). Helping others is certainly one way to honor God on Father's Day as well as feed our spirit and bring about inner joy.

How would the following kinds of activities bring about refreshment to you?

Physically: taking a nap, going for a walk, taking a bike ride

_____
_____
_____

Mentally: reading a book, going to an art museum, doing a crossword puzzle

_____
_____
_____

Emotionally: watching a positive movie, attending a ball game, playing miniature golf

_____
_____
_____

Spiritually: attending church, studying the Bible, praying, taking a drive to a quiet place to just breathe in fresh air and enjoy God's creation

_____
_____
_____

Different people find rest in different ways. Regular observance of the Sabbath—through worship and activities that brings about rest—will help develop the characteristic of faithfulness in the life of a Christian believer. Enjoy your Sabbath rest this week!

God, You certainly are Lord of the Sabbath. What a joy it is to take a day every week to worship You and to seek rest for my soul. Help me to make it not just a ritual but also a day that draws me more closely to You. In Jesus's name, amen.

Notes

1. The *NIV Study Bible* (Grand Rapids, MI: Zondervan, 1985), 1555, notes for Luke 8:19.

2. The *Book of Common Prayer* (New York: Oxford University Press, 1952), 301.

3. Brent Curtis and John Eldredge, *The Sacred Romance* (Nashville, TN: Thomas Nelson Publishers, 1997), p. 114.

4. Tim Keller, "Are Historic Christian Practices Still Relevant Today?" Q Ideas, 2014, accessed September 25, 2015, qideas.org/articles/wisdom-and-sabbath-rest.

WEEK SEVEN: TRAINING IN COMPASSION

SCRIPTURE MEMORY VERSE

"Love the Lord your God with all your heart and with all your soul and with all your mind and with all your strength." The second is this: "Love your neighbor as yourself." There is no commandment greater than these. Mark 12:30-31

Jesus's mission was to demonstrate the Father's compassionate love to a world that was trying to relegate God to fine print. The Jewish faith had been confined to figurative boxes of commandments, laws, regulations, and instructions. Spiritual holiness was marked by physical and behavioral perfection.

People tried to work out their faith by following Levitical regulations governing such things as cleanness of food, childbirth, infections, and more. They had to make the right kinds of offerings to atone for various kinds of offenses. But then came the *Word*, and that Word—Jesus—became the fulfillment of the Word of God. As He lived and breathed and taught on earth, He synthesized all the teachings of the Old Testament into a new standard: love.

One of the greatest pieces of understanding we can gain through our Personal Trainer, Jesus, is that He compassionately loved people. Certainly He loved His disciples and family, but He also greatly loved the common man and woman on the street. He noticed their hurts and needs. He empathized with them, spoke hope and encouragement into them, and demonstrated that compassion in tangible, life-changing ways. Additionally, because He wept, we know that He was not only the God-sent Word but also a man with human emotions.

—— DAY 1: SEE THE COMMONALITIES

Father, help me to truly notice the people around me during my day. Help me to take advantage of unique opportunities You provide to love them on Your behalf. In Jesus's name, amen.

One time when Jesus was teaching the people, a teacher of the Law asked Him to say which of the commandments was the greatest. Read Mark 12:28-34. How did

Jesus respond (see verses 29-31)?

_____

_____

_____

Turn to Exodus 20:1-17. How did Jesus synthesize the teaching of these Ten Commandments into two new ones?

_____

_____

_____

Clearly, Jesus knew love for God and love for others was at the heart of the Ten Commandments. As believers we become children of God—part of the same family—so we are not only neighbors but also people God calls His own. Think of someone who is a challenge for you. What commonalities do you share?

_____

_____

_____

Now write out a prayer, asking the Lord to build His compassion into you.

_____

_____

_____

Lord, I want to love You with all my heart, soul, mind, and strength. You are worthy of that love, and I want others to experience that kind of love from me. In Jesus's name, amen.

—— DAY 2: NOTICE OTHERS

Father, I do not want to miss opportunities to demonstrate Your compassion to others simply because I am in a busy fog. Help me to see others as You do. In Jesus's name, amen.

It would be difficult to show love toward others if we were self-absorbed and aware of only our own agenda. Compassionate people notice others' needs. Clearly, Jesus was observant and put other people's needs above His own—even when His healings jeopardized His own safety. Read Luke 6:6-11. Whom did Jesus see in the Temple with a physical need (see verse 6)? Despite the fact others are watching Him, what did He do (see verse 10)?

_____

_____

_____

Notice that Jesus saw the man in the first place. How must He have felt for the man?

_____

_____

_____

Read Luke 14:1-4. Whom did Jesus notice when He was invited for a meal at a Pharisee's house (see verse 2)? What did He do (see verse 4)?

_____

_____

_____

Jesus had been invited to the home of an *important* Jewish leader, and there would have been certain proprieties involved with touching a man who was ill (especially on the Sabbath). Why do you think Jesus chose to get involved?

_____

_____

_____

Why is it hard to notice the needs of those with whom we have contact during a typical day?

_____

_____

_____

What could you do to be more outwardly focused?

_____

_____

_____

Lord, You noticed the broken and lowly people wherever You went. Focus my eyes on others and their needs so I can develop Your compassion in my life. In Jesus's name, amen.

—— DAY 3: EMPATHIZE

Father, I love that prayer gives me insight and love for others. Develop compassion in me as I intercede for the needs of those around me. In Jesus's name, amen

We begin to develop Christ's compassion for others when we notice their needs, but we develop *empathy* for them when our hearts are touched. The word empathy comes from the Greek prefix *em*, which means "in," and *pathos*, which means "feeling." So, when we empathize with others, we have the ability to understand and share their feelings. Read Matthew 9:35-38. What three activities did Jesus do during His travels (see verse 35)?

_____

_____

_____

How were these three activities connected?

_____

_____

_____

How did Matthew describe the crowds of people (see verse 36)?

_____

_____

_____

To what did he compare them (see verse 36)?

_____

_____

_____

One expert reports, "When one sheep moves, the rest will follow, even if it is not a good idea. The flocking and following instinct of sheep is so strong that it caused the death of 400 sheep in 2006 in eastern Turkey. The sheep plunged to their death after one of the sheep tried to cross a 15-meter deep ravine, and the rest of the flock followed."[1] In Jesus's day there were no fences to contain sheep, so a shepherd

WEEK SEVEN TRAINING IN COMPASSION

had to guide them away from hazards and lead them to pastureland. When Jesus saw that the people were "like sheep without a shepherd," how did He respond (see verse 36)?

_____

_____

_____

What did Jesus explain to His disciples in verses 37-38? What do you think He felt was the deepest need of the people?

_____

_____

_____

Think of someone you know who needs Christ touch. What is that person's greatest need? How could you help him or her?

_____

_____

_____

Take a minute to pray for that person and for the opportunity to extend the touch of Jesus to him or her.

Lord, when You saw crowds of people, You did not simply see a sea of faces. Make my heart like Yours so I empathize with those You also love. In Jesus's name, amen.

—— DAY 4: ENCOURAGE

Father, words have such power. Just as You speak encouragement into my soul, I can choose to extend compassion and build up others with a kind word. In Jesus's name, amen.

John 3:16 may be the most famous verse that Jesus spoke: "For God so loved the world that he gave his one and only Son, that whoever believes in him shall not perish but have eternal life." However, some may not realize this statement was in response to questions from Nicodemus, who was a member of the Jewish ruling council. Read the full context in John 3:1-18. What did Nicodemus want to know (see verses 3-4)?

_____

_____

_____

Nicodemus came to Jesus at night, so his questions were probably not meant to trap Him. He addressed Christ as "rabbi," a term of respect, and said they knew He was from God because of the miracles He had performed (see verse 2). Jesus then taught Nicodemus how to have eternal life (see verses 5-6). But His words confused Nicodemus, because they probably changed what he thought was needed to have a relationship with God and experience eternal life. Jesus's words may have transformed Nicodemus's thinking (see John 7:50-51) and led him to be a Christ follower. What were Jesus's life-breathing words in verses 16-17?

_____

_____

_____

How must these words have affected Nicodemus?

_____

_____

_____

Who is someone you know who needs encouragement? What Scripture verse could enourage that person at this time?

_____

_____

_____

There are several ways to share an encouraging word: a visit, a phone call, a text message, an email. A special way to share compassion, though, is through a handwritten note, which can just take a few minutes. Share your love of Jesus with someone today.

Lord, You gave Your one and only Son, Jesus Christ, so I could have a relationship with You. Thank You for sending the Word of Life, the True Light of the world. In Jesus's name, amen.

—— DAY 5: EXTEND HELP

Father, Your Son demonstrated His love for people by helping them. Direct me to step out boldly in Christ's name and be Your hands and feet in the world. In Jesus's name, amen.

In 2007, a Muslim man named Hassan Askari took a beating on a New York subway on behalf of some Jewish women who were travelling together. The incident began when a group of thugs started harassing the women and their male friends by shouting, "Merry Christmas!" The male friends responded, "Happy Chanukah."

Askari, fearing for the women's safety, pushed one of the thugs away and was then attacked by the group. His actions gave one of the women's male friends time to pull the emergency brake on the train, which alerted officials of the trouble. The thugs beat up the 140-pound Askari, but he had no regrets. "I did what I thought was right," he said. "I did the best that I could to help."

In many ways, Askari is a modern-day Good Samaritan. In Jesus's time, the Samaritans were Jews who had assimilated with people who did not believe in God and did not practice or believe all the Scripture. The Jews viewed them as hated foreigners because of this and other differences between the groups.

Read Luke 10:25-37. When the expert in the law asked Jesus how to inherit eternal life, how did Jesus answer (see verse 27)?

_____

_____

_____

The expert then asked Jesus to define who was his neighbor. Most likely, the questioner wanted to know the exact boundaries for that definition—whether his "neighbor" was the man on the other side of his living wall or perhaps one or two walls beyond that. Through the parable Jesus defined the word neighbor for the expert and for all of us since.

The victim in Jesus's story was a man traveling from Jerusalem to Jericho. The trek was not an easy one. The first-century road was about eighteen miles long and descended from about 2,500 feet above to about 825 feet below sea level. The temperature shift was significant—from a Mediterranean climate to more of an African one that was dry until travelers reached Jericho (which was somewhat of an oasis). It was an arduous and dry trip—and one commonly frequented by bandits, who took advantage of the weary.[2] What happened to the man when he travelled from Jerusalem to Jericho (see verse 30)?

_____

_____

_____

How did each of the following people respond to the injured man (see verses 31-35)?

The Priest	
The Levite	
The Samaritan	

After hearing the parable, the expert in the law gave a definition of the word neighbor (see verse 37). What was that definition?

_____

_____

_____

The Good Samaritan in Jesus's parable demonstrated compassion, just as Hassan Askari did on the New York subway. What kinds of people today could be viewed as Samaritan-type figures? Who might be seen as an outcast of society?

_____

_____

_____

Compassionate people not only notice others' needs and empathize with them but also take action to make a difference in their lives. They demonstrate courage to defend and help those whom others shun. One organization that helps people in such sacrificial ways is Samaritan's Purse, which provides food, clothing, and other tangible gifts to people around the world who have suffered from natural disasters, persecution, and poverty. The organization derives its mission from the command Jesus gave to the expert in the law after telling him the parable of the Good Samaritan: "Go and do likewise" (Luke 10:37).[3] How could you follow Jesus's command this week to help someone you know who is in need?

_____

_____

_____

Jesus, You healed people of physical afflictions and gave Your life for me on the cross. May I be a vehicle for Your compassion by extending a hand to someone in need. In Your name, amen.

—— DAY 6: REFLECTION AND APPLICATION

Father, Your Son demonstrated His love for people by helping them. Direct me to step out boldly in Christ's name and be Your hands and feet in the world today. In Jesus's name, amen.

A Hebrew expression that precedes this week's memory verse is, "Hear, O Israel: The LORD our God, the LORD is one" (Deuteronomy 6:4). Joined with Deuteronomy 6:5, it is known as the *Shema*, which means "hear" in Hebrew. Devout Jews in Jesus's day recited this statement of faith every morning and evening, and Jewish people today still begin their synagogue services by reciting it. To the Shema, Jesus added "and with all your mind," and then dovetailed a synthesis of the last six commandments as the second greatest commandment: "Love your neighbor as yourself." Clearly, one of our most important tasks is demonstrating love for God and love toward others.

What does that kind of love look like? When we love God with all our *heart*, we focus our emotional center on Him so that our greatest delight is spending time with Him. Our soul-filled love for God comes from our very essence—that eternal, life-breathing force within us that focuses our conscience in a heavenward direction so our spirit wants the things of God. When we love the Lord with all our *mind*, we intellectually desire to know more about God and want to satisfy our curiosity about who is the Creator and Redeemer. Loving God with all our *strength* means we are not half-hearted about our relationship with God. Instead, we put our whole self into the work the Lord has for us—serving and loving His people.

Joseph DeVeuster, also known as Father Damien, was a man who loved and served people in just this way. Born into a Flemish family in Belgium, he became a priest in the Catholic Church. In 1873, he was the first to volunteer to help those suffering from Hansen's disease, also known as leprosy, on the Hawaiian island of Molokai. There he attended to the medical needs of more than 800 lepers. He also built a church, homes, furniture, and 600 coffins for those who died—and dug their graves as well.

At the time it was believed that leprosy was highly contagious, so the Hawaiian kingdom quarantined those who had the disease—including many children—and created a leper colony on Molokai. Father Damien became especially concerned for these children and organized the construction of orphanage buildings. When provisions for the care of those in the colony became meager, Father Damien advocated for additional provisions.

Although it has since been discovered that leprosy is not as contagious as once thought, Father Damien did contract the disease twelve years after his arrival and died from it at age 49. It was his compassion that led him to volunteer to minister at the leper colony, and it was his compassion to mix closely with the people that led to his death. He explained this by saying, "I make myself a leper with the lepers to gain all to Jesus Christ."[4] Father Damien's love for God was manifested in his sacrificial love for a society viewed as unlovely outcasts.

Through this study you have been challenging yourself to make changes in the four areas of your life: physical, mental, emotional, and spiritual. Similarly, through the Greatest Commandment, Jesus challenges you to love God in four different ways. This week, consider how your love for God could be demonstrated in compassionate ways toward those in your First Place for Health group or with others close to you.

Lord, it takes everything I have to love You with the love You deserve. Today, I pray that You would develop in me the love that You have for people. In Jesus's name, amen.

—— DAY 7: REFLECTION AND APPLICATION

Father, in Your great compassion You sent Jesus to be a servant to all—through His life, His service, and His death. Develop a servant heart in me so that my example lives up to Your name. In Jesus's name, amen.

Jesus demonstrated compassion in many ways. He fed the masses when they were hungry. He healed the sick and demon-possessed. He reassured His disciples that He would never leave them nor forsake them. Again and again we see that our Personal Trainer saw the needs of people and quickly moved to action. However, the Gospels only record Him weeping twice.

The first time was when His friend Lazarus died (see John 11). In this instance, Jesus didn't weep with the news of Lazarus's death but when he saw Lazarus's sister Mary (and others) weeping and saying, "Lord, if you had been here, my brother would not have died" (verse 32). Jesus wept because she was heartbroken—and *then* He went to the tomb and resurrected Lazarus. Broken hearts moved Jesus to compassionate tears.

The second time Jesus wept was when He approached Jerusalem for the last time before His crucifixion. Luke wrote, "As he approached Jerusalem and saw the city, he wept over it" (19:41). The Greek word for wept indicates a loud expression of grief, especially in mourning.[5] Jesus's eyes, which had swept over the city, moved His heart, and His heart broke over a city filled with people who would reject Him and scream, "Crucify him! Crucify him!" Lost souls also moved Jesus to tears.

Read Luke 19:41-44. What did Jesus wish the people had known (see verse 42)?

_____

_____

_____

Why do you think Jesus said this peace was hidden from the people's eyes?

_____

_____

_____

In Luke 19:43-44, Jesus prophesied about a time when the city would fall to foreign invasion, with mass destruction and death. This occurred just 40 years later in AD 70, when the Jews revolted against a Roman procurator who seized silver from the Temple to subsidize his tax revenues. Jewish zealots took over the Roman fortress at Masada, which propelled bold solidarity in Jerusalem and led to an all-out war against the Romans. Eventually, the Roman battering rams and ballistae—rock-throwing machines—broke down the city's walls.[6]

The Temple was completely destroyed, fulfilling Jesus's prophesy in Luke 19:44: "They will not leave one stone on another." Those who had refused to believe in Christ had worked with Roman authorities to bring about His death, and now, less than a century later, the city had fallen to those very Romans authorites. Jesus knew all that would be ahead for those who rejected Him—and He wept for them.

For whom do you weep? Who within your area of influence do not know Christ? This week, pray that they will come to know the Savior who would weep for them—and who gave His life on the cross so they might have eternal life.

Lord, Your Son, Jesus, is the ultimate example of compassion. He saw the immediate needs of people, but He also saw their greatest need—to have a personal relationship with You. Stir my heart daily to pray for those who need You. In Jesus's name, amen.

Notes

1. Susan Schoenian, "Sheep 201: A Beginner's Guide to Raising Sheep," June 18, 2011, accessed October 1, 2015, http://www.sheep101.info/201/behavior.html.

2. "From Jerusalem to Jericho," American Bible Society, accessed October 6, 2015, http://bibleresources.americanbible.org/resource/from-jerusalem-to-jericho.

3. Samaritan's Purse, "About Us," accessed October 6, 2015, www.samaritanspurse.org.

4. "Father Damien," Kalaupapa National Historical Park, Hawai'i, National Park Service, accessed November 18, 2015, http://www.nps.gov/kala/learn/historyculture/damien.htm.

5. W.E. Vine, An Expository Dictionary of New Testament Words (Old Tappan, NJ: Fleming H. Revell Company, 1966), 206.

6. "A.D. 70 Titus Destroys Jerusalem," Christianity Today, October 1, 1990, accessed October 20, 2015, http://www.christianitytoday.com/ch/1990/issue28/2808.html?start=1.

WEEK EIGHT: TRAINING IN COMPOSURE

SCRIPTURE MEMORY VERSE
My kingdom is not of this world. John 18:36

Jesus's walk to the cross was one of composure, in which He demonstrated a calmness that seemingly was not of this world. We see in John 18–19 that He submitted to arrest without a fight and without attempting to flee. When soldiers took him to Annas, the high priest, He answered questions simply about His disciples and His teachings. When He was taken to Pilate, the Roman governor, He said, "My kingdom is not of this world." With the shadow of the cross before Him, He maintained a tranquil strength because He knew that on the other side of suffering, His Father was waiting for Him.

We can also have faith through suffering because our suffering can also have purpose. L.B. Cowman writes in *Streams in the Desert*, "In order to have a sympathetic God, we must have a suffering Savior, for true sympathy comes from understanding another person's hurt by suffering the same affliction. Therefore we cannot help others who suffer without paying a price ourselves, because afflictions are the cost we pay for our ability to sympathize. Those who wish to help others must first suffer. If we wish to rescue others, we must be willing to face the cross; experiencing the greatest happiness in life through ministering to others is impossible without drinking the cup Jesus drank and without submitting to the baptism He endured."[1]

Just as Christ demonstrated composure during that most difficult time of His life, He also had willpower and self-discipline in other circumstances. From His example we can find inspiration for godly living as we face daily challenges—and even great suffering—so others may see how our faith makes a difference in even the toughest of times.

—— DAY 1: EXERCISE PATIENCE
Father, develop the quality of patience in me so I do not rashly respond in the face of criticism or on the heels of suffering. Point me daily toward Your face. In Jesus's name, amen.

Life is stress-filled. Our work demands seemingly impossible deadlines. Neighbors are not neighborly. Friends disappoint us. Family members bicker and squabble. Even worse, disease, aging, and our weight zap our strength and layer worry upon worry. In response we might lose our cool and strike out with worried words or caustic criticism. However, instead of rushing ahead with words and actions, Jesus would say, "Abide in me." Read John 15:1-8. To what does Jesus compare Himself and His heavenly Father (see verse 1)?

_____

_____

_____

Fill in the following blanks from verses 4-7:

_____ in me, as I also will _____ in you. No branch can bear fruit by itself; it must _____ in the vine. Neither can you bear fruit unless you _____ in me. I am the vine; you are the branches. If you _____ in me and I in you, you will bear much fruit; apart from me you can do nothing. If you do not _____ in me, you are like a branch that is thrown away and withers; such branches are picked up, thrown into the fire and burned. If you _____ in me and my words _____ in you, ask whatever you wish, and it will be done for you.

According to these verses, when a person remains (or abides) in Christ, what happens to that person? What happens if the person chooses not to abide in Christ?

_____

_____

_____

South African minister Andrew Murray experienced a difficult time in his life when he lost his voice and was unable to preach for two years. He also suffered from a serious horse-cart injury, which prevented him from travelling to speak around the world. However, his daughter later wrote that he developed a dear relationship with God in prayer because of this disability.[2] One of the fruits of this period was his work *Abide in Christ*, in which he shared, "Each time your attention is free to occupy itself with the thought of Jesus—whether it be with time to think and pray, or only for a few passing seconds—let your first thought be to say: *Now, at this moment, I do abide in Jesus*."[3]

As Christians, we can conquer our emotions by choosing to remember our position with our Savior. We are a branch of the Vine, which is Jesus. Sometimes, in the heat of a stress-filled day or the busyness of our schedule, we forget who we are. During such times, we can take a sacred pause to hear God's voice and sense His nudge "this way" or "that way."

This requires *patience*. Some may say, "Oh, don't pray for patience! You don't want the life lesson God might give you!" Yet patience is indeed a fruit of the spirit (see Galatians 5:22). It is a quality we can develop by making choices to wait for God's assurance of His best, listen for His direction, read the Bible, meditate on Scripture, and choose the quality of composure. As we patiently wait, we can choose to avoid assumptions when tense situations arise. We can research, ask questions, be a good listener to others, and find out the truth God would have us see behind a veil of confusion or frustration. As we do so, we will "bear much fruit" (John 15:5).

What would it look like in each of the four areas if your life began to bear much fruit?

Physically	
Emotionally	
Mentally	
Spiritually	

Lord, even through the ups and downs I can take a sacred pause, breathe, and remember that the Gardener of My Soul is still at work in my life. In Jesus's name, amen.

—— DAY 2: STAY POSITIVE

Father, I know I can always look to You for comfort when others disappoint me. Because You pressed on, I can as well! In Jesus's name, amen.

As "Mariel" was nearing the end of her long tenure as a high school teacher, athletic director, and principal, I asked her, "How do you stay so positive? Students, parents, and even coaches parade into your office and complain and give you a hard time. What is your secret for keeping your composure when they are mean-spirited?"

Mariel said, "I simply refuse to be offended." She went on to explain she had learned that people will always have their own ideas about what is right and wrong, so she decided years ago not to take comments personally. While it was challenging for her to face insults and name-calling, she kept her composure and kept a positive attitude.

Even Jesus had to face the betrayal of friends. His disciple Judas turned Him over to authorities. Peter denied knowing Him. Most of the other disciples slipped into the shadows at His crucifixion. Read Mark 14:27-31. Whom did Jesus say would desert him (see verse 27)?

_____
_____
_____

How did Peter respond (see verse 29)?

_____
_____
_____

What were the next three responses . . .

From Jesus (v. 30)	
From Peter (v. 31)	
From the others (v.31)	

Read Mark 14:66-72. How did Peter respond to . . .

The servant girl (vv.66-68)	
The servant girl (vv. 69-70)	
The crowd (vv. 70-71)	

After Peter's third denial, he heard the rooster crow and remembered Jesus had predicted his denial. How did he then respond (see verse 72)? Why would he respond in that way?

_____

_____

_____

Despite the betrayal of His closest friends, Jesus calmly responded "I am" when asked if He was the Son of the Blessed One (Mark 14:62) and "yes, it is as you say" when asked if He was the king of the Jews (Mark 15:2). He did not allow His emotions to take over. Ultimately, He knew that in the face of seeming injustice, His Father was in control—and that was enough. Similarly, when life seems out of control, you can do the following:

1. **Refuse to be offended.** Everyone has his or her ideas, and those ideas need not sidetrack you from what you know to be true.
2. **Recognize you cannot control what others say and do, and you cannot control all circumstances.** However, you can, with God's help, control your reactions to those people and circumstances.
3. **Think about why a situation might upset you and determine what might be the root of your annoyance.** Are you jealous of someone? Do you feel you are being overlooked? Do you feel you are being treated unjustly?
4. **Pray and trust God for the outcome.** It is amazing how God can either change a situation or change our hearts about it.

Lord, You always have my best interests in mind. Help me choose not to be offended by others and choose to be Your example of grace. In Jesus's name, amen.

—— DAY 3: ACCEPT THE SITUATION

Father, I want to represent You well and please You. When others see me hard-pressed on all sides, may my words and actions bring glory to Your name! In Jesus's name, amen.

As Christians, we know God is *sovereign* in our lives. The word sovereign comes from the Old French *soverain*, which comes from the Latin *super* (meaning "above" or "over") and regnum (meaning "rex" or "king"). So, when we say God is sovereign, we are saying He is the king above all else. His plan for us is perfect, His guidance is just right, and the circumstances He allows will draw us more closely to Him. When we cling to those truths, we respond to challenging circumstances in a Christ-like manner, knowing our Father God has the bigger picture in mind. Read John 13:18-30. How did Jesus refer to the person who would betray Him (see verse 18)?

_____

_____

_____

Sharing a meal indicated a close familial relationship or friendship. How did Jesus feel about this betrayal in the making (see verse 21)?

_____

_____

_____

How would you feel if a friend falsely accused you and turned you over to legal authorities?

_____

_____

_____

The disciples were confused at Jesus's remarks, so Peter prompted John to say, "Lord, who is it?" (verse 25). How did Jesus respond in the next verses? What did Jesus say to the one who would betray Him?

_____

_____

_____

The disciples still did not understand what Jesus was indicating. Why might they have been confused about this (see verses 28-29)?

_____

_____

_____

Have you experienced a time when you felt betrayed by someone you loved? Did that situation sideline you emotionally so you did not respond well? Explain what happened.

_____

_____

_____

Thinking back on that incident, how might Jesus have responded if in that situation?

_____

_____

_____

Lord, nothing happens without the filter of Your perfect will for my life. Thus, I will praise You, thank You, and give You glory for every episode of every day. In Jesus's name, amen.

—— DAY 4: SEEK GOD'S HELP

Father, I want to be so connected to You that I see Your hand in all aspects of my life! In Jesus's name, amen.

After Jesus passed the dipped bread to His betrayer, He spent more time with the rest of the disciples, teaching them and comforting them (see John 14–16). At that point, He knew His time was short and His arrest was imminent. So He did what we should do if we want to develop the trait of composure: *pray.* Read Jesus's chapter-long prayer in John 17. How did He address God (see verses 1, 5, 11, 21, 24, 25)?

_____

_____

_____

In verse 1, Jesus spoke frankly with His Father and said, "Father, the hour has come." What do you think He meant by that? To what was He resigned?

_____

_____

_____

Jesus next took care of final business on earth with three different groups of requests. What is at least one request Jesus made to His Father in each group?

Prayers for Himself (vv. 1-5)	
Prayers for disciples (vv. 6-19)	
Prayers for all believers (vv. 20-26)	

Notice in the last group of prayer requests that Jesus was praying for *us*. Which of those requests do you take to heart most dearly?

_____
_____
_____

Jesus looked to God before facing the toughest day of His life. Prayer is not a way to wimp out in times of trial but is the best problem-solving strategy. Through prayer, we leave our problems in God's hands and ask Him to work through us. We pray for the other person involved in the situation, and sometimes that can help us see the situation from that person's point of view. God takes care of the details that are out of our control. What prayer requests do you have for a tough situation you or another loved one is facing?

_____
_____
_____

Lord God, I love that I can come to You, hand over my struggles, and watch You work. Thank You for taking the pressure off me and assuring me You are at work! In Jesus's name, amen.

—— DAY 5: REMAIN FEARLESS

Father, as waves crash around me, You are the stilling factor in my storm. I will keep my eyes on You and not be afraid. In Jesus's name, amen.

Jesus did not run from His persecutors but fearlessly walked into their hands. Read John 18:1-11. What person met Jesus in the olive grove (see verse 2)?

_____
_____
_____

Who was with him? How were they prepared to confront Jesus (see verse 3)?

_____
_____
_____

We learn from verse 4 that Jesus knew what was going to happen. So why did He walk straight into that situation?

_____

_____

_____

When the group indicated they were looking for "Jesus of Nazareth," how did He respond (see verse 5)?

_____

_____

_____

One commentator wrote, "They came to arrest a meek peasant and instead were met in the dim light by a majestic person."[4] Fearless people stun others, as the story of Louise and Nathan Degrafinried shows. This couple was confronted in their Tennessee home by an escaped convict weilding a gun. When Nathan went to ready their truck for the man, the convict aimed his shotgun at Louise. She calmly said, "Young man, I'm a Christian lady. We don't have any violence in this house. This is God's house. Put that gun down."

After another warning, he said, "Lady, I'm so hungry. I haven't eaten in three days." Louise fixed him breakfast, said grace over the food, and prepared a solution to soothe his sore throat. The criminal told Louise she reminded him of his grandmother, who was dead. Louise replied, "Well, I love you, and I'm not dead. Jesus loves you, too." A short time later she talked the young man into giving himself up.[5] Jesus likewise talked sense into the armed detachment who had come to arrest Him. What did He request (see verses 8-9)?

_____

_____

_____

Then what did Peter do (see verse 10)?

_____

_____

_____

There is a difference between being fearless for God and lashing out emotionally. Jesus was prayed up and knew what His Father wanted Him to do. Peter was reacting without thinking, as he often did. How did Jesus respond to Peter's action (see verse 11)?

_____

_____

_____

How have you responded with an impulsive "Peter-ism" when faced with something difficult?

_____

_____

_____

Thinking back on that situation, what might have been a better response?

_____

_____

_____

Christians have received grace, and we are called to respond gracefully in tense situations. Here are some suggestions to follow:

1. **Vent appropriately.** Don't gossip about the people involved but write a letter that you do not send. The simple act of putting something down and then tearing it up can help you resolve hurt.
2. **Be accountable for any part you have played.** Owning up to your responsibility can help defuse how the issue could play out negatively.
3. **Stave off a fight-or-flight tendency.** Running from the problem will not help, and fighting will only escalate matters to a tougher situation.
4. **Fearlessly face what is ahead.** Know that your Sovereign God is in control.

Father, Jesus faced an armed crowd with dignity, grace, and composure. Develop those qualities in me so I can face my future fearlessly. In Jesus's name, amen.

—— DAY 6: REFLECTION AND APPLICATION
Father, when life is a mess, You are still with me, comforting, guiding, and directing me. I want to be aware of Your presence so I can respond with composure. In Jesus's name, amen.

Sometimes we overreact to negative triggers in our lives. These triggers could be a sarcastic comment or a rude driver or something as simple as the kitchen left in a mess. It is challenging to retain our composure during such times, but it can be done—especially when we consider that, ultimately, our kingdom is not of this world. The hurts and difficulties we face are temporal because the comfort and joy of heaven is just around the corner.

Jesus faced cruelties at His crucifixion—incidents that could have made Him lash out in anger. In Matthew 27:27-31, we read the soldiers stripped Him, put a scarlet robe on Him, and set a crown of thorns on His head. They put a staff in His hand and mocked Him by saying, "Hail, king of the Jews!" (verse 29). Then they spit on Him and struck Him. Despite the cruelties—any of which could cause a person to lose control—Jesus remained composed.

After Jesus told Pilate that He was king of the Jews (see verse 11), Jesus said, "But now my kingdom is from another place" (John 18:36). He was aware of who He was. While part of His self-composure rested in this identity, another part of Him was fully man who experienced the same kinds of struggles that we do—disappointments, hurts, and even betrayal by friends. However, God was able to fulfill His plan through His Son because Jesus did not let earthly distractions trigger reactions that would have led Him down a different path.

As you grow in your faith, you will become more aware of triggers that kick off bad attitudes and responses. These negative triggers can make you react with sarcasm, bad language, overeating, depression, gossip, and avoidance of others. However, now that you have been studying about Christ's composure this week, what is one change you will make to respond to negative triggers in a more godly manner?

_____

_____

_____

Lord, I am thankful that I have the opportunity to live out life on earth with You. Keep my eyes focused on Your bigger picture for my life. In Jesus's name, amen.

—— DAY 7: REFLECTION AND APPLICATION

Father, I know there are times when I need to take a stand for Your sake. I trust that You will give me Your words and the courage to speak them. In Jesus's name, amen.

In Jesus' day, when people traveled to the Temple in Jerusalem, they were often unable to take animals with them that they needed for the sacrifices. So merchants set up shop tables in the courtyard for the purpose of selling animals to travelers. There were also moneychangers there—people who exchanged foreign coins for those that would be accepted at the Temple. This seems a rather innocent practice, except that extortion was common.

Matthew tells us that when Jesus entered the Temple, He chased out the people who were buying and selling there. He even overturned the tables of the moneychangers and the benches of those selling doves. Jesus then referred to Isaiah 56:7, in which the LORD said the Temple was a house of prayer. However, when Jesus quoted it, He referred to the Temple as "My house" and said the people were making it a "den of robbers" (see Matthew 21:12-17).

Clearly, this deviates from what we would consider an example of composure. However, the sellers and moneychangers had set up their businesses in the Court of Gentiles. God had intended for all people to be able to worship in the Temple, but this commercialism was keeping them from gaining access to their place of worship. Jesus simply demonstrated that no one should be impeded from openly worshiping God.

In Mark's account, we read that the chief priests and teachers of the law observed the incident. But instead of arresting Jesus for causing a disturbance, they "feared him, because the whole crowd was amazed at his teaching" (11:18) and began looking for a way to kill Him. It appears Jesus was enforcing God's laws in clearing out the Temple. He was also threatening the religious leaders who had not only tolerated these practices but also probably profited from them.

The blind and the lame came to Jesus for healing. Children shouted, "Hosanna to the Son of David" (Matthew 21:15). We can see that the weakest of society—the blind, the lame, the children—did not view Jesus as a madman who was a threat to people's personal safety. In the same way, God will give you wisdom, clarity, and decisiveness when you need to take a stand for your faith or when others are being mistreated. This week, think about a principle you could draw from this incident. In what situations *would* it be appropriate to react with emotion?

Lord, I know You will give me wisdom and boldness to speak Your truth when Your name is at stake. I trust You for protecting me in times of challenge. In Jesus's name, amen.

Notes

1. L.B. Cowman, *Streams in the Desert* (Grand Rapids, MI: Zondervan, 1997), 279.

2. Janet Holm McHenry, *PrayerStreaming* (Colorado Springs, CO: WaterBrook, 2005), 78.

3. Andrew Murray, *Abide in Christ* (Fort Washington, PA: Christian Literature Crusade, 1972), 87.

4. The *NIV Study Bible* (Grand Rapids, MI: Zondervan, 185), 1631, footnote for John 18:6.

5. Robert J. Morgan, Stories, *Illustrations, and Quotes* (Nashville, TN: Thomas Nelson, 2000), 300-301.

WEEK NINE: TRAINING IN INTEGRITY

SCRIPTURE MEMORY VERSE

If anyone, then, who knows the good they ought to do and doesn't do it, it is sin for them. James 4:17

The *San Francisco Chronicle* once asked its readers, "If you found $500,000 in the street and knew it belonged to someone else, but discovered that legally you could keep it, would you?" San Francisco Giants relief pitcher Jeremy Affeldt did not. When his contract was renegotiated in 2010, he was set to earn $4 million, but due to a clerical error, the contract read $4.5 million. Both the Giants and Affeldt signed the contract without noticing the mistake.

When Affeldt was made aware of it, he consulted his agent, a Players Association representative, and the Giants' assistant general manager, all of whom agreed he could legally keep the money. But Affeldt shocked the baseball world by giving back the $500,000 to the Giants organization. When asked why, the devout Christian father of three said he didn't feel easy about profiting from the error. "I won't sleep well at night knowing I took that money, because every time I open my paycheck I'll know it's not right," he said. This led him to return the money and get the contract rewritten.[1]

Integrity—synonymous with *character*—is the quality of having moral and ethical strength. It is doing the right thing for the right reason, even when no one is watching. When we do the right thing, practice what we preach, and are honest in our day-to-day dealings with others, we will be people of integrity.

—— DAY 1: RELY ON THE SPIRIT

Father, I want to live a life of integrity because the world watches as I live out my life before others. Help me make right decisions with the guidance of Your Spirit. In Jesus's name, amen.

Integrity was another characteristic that Christ possessed. He was honest and good, and led a life of authenticity. He proclaimed the truth with sincerity, adhered to a pattern of good works, and modeled a standard of completeness by which all Christians are compared. Yet following Jesus could be a seemingly impossible task without the help that God provided. Read John 14:15-21. What did Jesus say the Father would provide to believers (see verse 16)?

_____

_____

_____

What is another name for this advocate (see verse 17)?

_____

_____

_____

Where would the Holy Spirit live (see verse 17)?

_____

_____

_____

Jesus knew His departure could leave the disciples feeling powerless to live, teach, and preach. So He promised He would not leave them as orphans on earth. Read Acts 1:4-8. Just before Jesus ascended to heaven, what did He tell the disciples to do (see verse 4)?

_____

_____

_____

What did Jesus say the disciples would receive when the Spirit came (see verse 8)? For what purpose was this to be used?

_____

_____

_____

Read Acts 2:1-17. What happened on the Day of Pentecost (see verses 2-4)?

_____

_____

_____

The Holy Spirit empowered the believers to do works they were previously unable to do: speak in other languages, prophesy, and preach. What did Peter immediately do (see verse 14)?

_____

_____

_____

When you professed faith in Jesus Christ, the Holy Spirit began empowering you to live a life of integrity. How can the Spirit help you with your First Place for Health goals this week?

_____

_____

_____

Lord God, with the help of Your Spirit, I can make choices that will bring honor to Your name and inspire others to learn why my faith makes a difference in my life. In Jesus's name, amen.

—— DAY 2: STUDY THE WORD

Father, guide me as I study the Bible. Reveal insights to me and help me to apply them to my life so that others will see You in me. In Jesus's name, amen.

Christians are always measured against the principles in God's Word. We are expected to do the right thing for the right reason—whether someone is watching or not. Certainly, God has forgiven us of our sins—past, present, and future—but if we want others to see God in us, we need to be a consistent student of God's Word. A good place to start is the Gospels, in which we read what Jesus taught about who He was, how we can choose eternal life with Him, how to love God and our neighbor, and how to live a holy life. First, read the following verses in John and fill in the blanks about who Jesus claimed to be.

John 10:30: "_____ and the _____ are _____."

John 10:36: "Why then do you accuse of me of blasphemy because I said, '_____ am _____ _____'?"

John 10:38: "The _____ is in _____, and _____ in the _____."

According to these verses, what is Jesus's relationship to God the Father?

_____

_____

_____

Next, fill in the blanks in these verses about how Jesus taught we can have eternal life:

John 3:3: "Very truly I tell you, no one can see the _____ of _____ unless they are _____ _____."

John 3:16: "For _____ so loved the _____ that he gave his one and only _____, that whoever _____ in him shall not perish but have _____ _____."

John 3:18: "Whoever _____ in him is not _____."

According to these verses, how does one obtain eternal life?

_____

_____

_____

Now again read Matthew 22:36-40, in which Jesus taught about love. What are the two most important laws in the Bible, according to Jesus?

_____

_____

_____

Many of Jesus's teachings were related to how to live rightly—to matters of integrity. One of His teachings relates to the value of a person's word. Read Matthew 5:33-37. What did Jesus teach about making oaths, which were vows based on God's name (see verses 34-36)?

_____

_____

_____

How would you summarize Jesus's teaching in verse 37?

_____

_____

_____

People of integrity are good for their word, so when we make a commitment, it is important to keep that commitment. Typical commitments could include deadlines at work, ministry responsibilities at church, and volunteerism for a school organization or community group. Is this an area in which you struggle? Explain your response.

_____

_____

_____

Studying the Bible—particularly the life of Christ—can help you become a more consistently committed Christ follower. As you study the Bible daily, the truth of God's Word will permeate your mind, soul, and heart, and help you make choices that testify to the power of God. This will enable you to not only be a person of your word but also of God's Word.

Lord, as I read and study Your Word, may I breathe in its principles and show others that my commitment to You is borne out in how I live every day. In Jesus's name, amen.

—— DAY 3: VALUE PEOPLE

Father, You accept and embrace me as Your own. I will extend that same kind of grace to others—whether they bear Your name or not. In Jesus's name, amen.

Jesus demonstrated integrity in His relationships with others. He did not favor those in power, cater to the wealthy, or choose disciples from the elite. Instead, He extended love to those in the lower echelons of society who could have potentially damaged His status with authorities. Read Luke 14:12-14. Why did Jesus say to the host that he should not invite friends, relatives, and rich neighbors to a luncheon or dinner (see verses 13-14)?

_____

_____

_____

Certainly, it's not wrong to invite friends and family to our home to socialize and share a meal. Jesus was simply teaching that because people of all kinds will be in heaven, we need to look past our natural social boundaries and get to know all kinds of people. Another group we might encounter in heaven are those we view as enemies. Read Matthew 5:43-48. A law in Leviticus instructed, "Do not seek revenge or bear a grudge against anyone among your people, but love your neighbor as yourself. I am the LORD" (19:18). Apparently, the Pharisees viewed the phrase "among your people" as a way out of loving their enemies. How did Jesus flip that interpretation (see Matthew 5:44)?

_____
_____
_____

What are some reasons Jesus listed for loving our enemies (see verses 45-48)?

_____
_____
_____

How might praying for an enemy—or even doing a kindness for that person—change the relationship?

_____
_____
_____

Another way Jesus mixed up social prejudices involved how He treated children and women (see Mark 10:13-16). John Ortberg notes the longest conversation Jesus had in Scripture was not with a man but with a woman—the Samaritan woman at the well (see John 4). "This woman was poor; she had to draw her own water. Jesus was saying: 'I know you. I know you're a woman, a Samaritan. Your life is very hard. I know your story. I care about you.' This rabbi sat at a well and engaged in a deep, theological, personal discussion about this woman's relationship with God. He took seriously her mind and opinions and questions."[2] Jesus also associated with the diseased and was known as "a friend of tax collectors and sinners" (Matthew 11:19). How could you demonstrate the love of Christ to others who might not normally be in your social circles?

_____
_____
_____

Lord, thank You for nudging me to get out of my comfort zone and extend Your grace to the least of these. Help me see others as future citizens of Your kingdom. In Jesus's name amen.

—— DAY 4: AVOID HYPOCRISY

Father, I know hypocrisy can be a stumbling block to others embracing a Christian faith. Help me be conscious of my actions, as I am Your ambassador here on earth. In Jesus's name, amen.

While none of us is perfect, and we are bound to make mistakes, we should make conscious decisions that represent Christ well. Everything matters. The word *hypocrisy* comes from Greek origins that mean "play acting" or "playing a part." How is being hypocritical like playing a part?

_____

_____

_____

Read Luke 6:37-42. What three actions did Jesus instruct us not to do (see verse 37)? What actions should we do instead (see verses 37-38)?

_____

_____

_____

What could be the relationship between forgiving and giving?

_____

_____

_____

How do we benefit by giving to others (see verse 38)? How could giving to someone we have forgiven help us to forget the original offense?

_____

_____

_____

Christ's whole purpose in coming to earth was to provide a way for forgiveness of our sins. So, when we are judgmental toward others, we are condemning those people whom Jesus came to save. How does God say He views people who judge others (see verse 37)?

_____

_____

_____

WEEK NINE TRAINING IN INTEGRITY

How is being judgmental like being blind (see verses 39-40)?

_____

_____

_____

Why might others find judgmental people hypocritical (see verses 41-42)?

_____

_____

_____

What does gossip have to do with these critical, judgmental attitudes? How could gossip keep others from pursuing a relationship with Christ?

_____

_____

_____

In Luke 6:39-40, Jesus taught that everyone who is fully trained will be like his teacher. Just as an athlete finds inspiration in his or her personal trainer at a gym or on a playing field, we can study and apply the teachings of Jesus to our own lives—and live free of critical and hypocritical attitudes that would otherwise keep us from growing more like Jesus every day. Take a minute to do some reflection about potentially hypocritical behaviors or words you have had. Write a short prayer here, asking God to help your walk match your talk in this specific area.

_____

_____

_____

Jesus, Your life spotlessly reflected Your holiness. Help me not to flail about blindly and misdirect others but instead point them to You with consistent behavior. In Jesus's name, amen.

—— DAY 5: PURSUE EXCELLENCE

Father, doing my best brings honor to You. May my life shine in the darkness around me in such a way that others are drawn to You through me. In Jesus's name, amen.

We serve a God of excellence. When He created the world and everything in it, after each act of creation He said, "It is good" (see Genesis 1:4, 10, 12, 18, 21, 25). Think about the design of nature. Snow-capped mountains cradling the clouds. Rivers winding snakelike through canyons and valleys. Layers of trees texturizing the landscape. Bursts of flora providing a finishing pop. Each day we have the opportunity to continue God's creative process by bringing excellence to our work—whether we do that in the home or at a job. Read Matthew 5:13-16. In this passage, Jesus used three metaphors. To what did He compare believers (see verse 13)?

_____

_____

_____

How can everyday salt make our lives better?

_____

_____

_____

How might believers demonstrate a figurative saltiness to their faith and behavior?

_____

_____

_____

If believers do not have that figurative saltiness, what is their value to God's kingdom (see verse 13)? Why would that be?

_____

_____

_____

What are the second and third metaphors that Jesus used to compare believers (see verse 14)?

_____

_____

_____

Turn off the lights in one of the rooms of your home. Then turn on one lamp and raise it up toward the ceiling. As you raise the lamp, how does that affect the lighting in the room?

_____

_____

_____

What did Jesus mean, then, about being the light of the world—a city on a hill?

_____
_____
_____

What is the effect of shining a Christ-like example (see verse 16)?

_____
_____
_____

Excellence—shining light—is offering the best of ourselves to God as we serve with our talents, time, and treasure. As Christians, we are designed to do excellence because we have the touch of the Creator within us and can tap into His creative resources of intellect and inspiration. Pursuit of excellence honors God and inspires others to do so as well. Perfection is unachievable—pursuing it can paralyze us in our tracks—but loving God so much that we simply want to please and honor Him makes work meaningful and effective.

We hear the expression, "When you do a job, you do your best!" Yet if we attempt to do our best in every role in our lives—if we try to be the best parent, the best spouse, the best friend, the best co-worker, the best ministry leader, the best volunteer—we might find it is almost impossible. The best way to approach each day is to learn to do our best moment by moment and trust God for His grace to help us in our pursuit of excellence.

Jesus, You set an example of how to live a purposeful, meaningful life. Guide me each day so I may live a life of integrity that shines a light to those in the darkness. In Jesus's name, amen.

—— DAY 6: REFLECTION AND APPLICATION
Father, I know that Your Spirit nudges me daily to do the right thing. There must be thousands of ways that You have protected me and helped me be a positive influence—and I am thankful for Your sovereign hand in my life. In Jesus's name, amen.

Do you have regrets about your life? We all make mistakes. We all have intentions to do good but fail to follow through on those intentions. Sometimes, as mentioned earlier this week, our walk does not match our talk. However, as our memory verse in James 4:17 states, when it is clear God has a work for us to do and we choose not to do it, we are acting in sin.

However, all is not a lost cause. We can recognize our mistakes and determine to move past them toward transformation in our lives. As mature, Christ-like individuals, we can examine our past, think about the poor choices we made, acknowledge them as mistakes, and decide to do better the next time God whispers, "Do this good thing." Even the evangelist Billy Graham, when reflecting back on his life, found that he would have done some things differently if he could have had a do-over. He wrote:

> I'd spend more time at home with my family, and I'd study more and preach less. I wouldn't have taken so many speaking engagements, including some of the things I did over the years that I probably didn't really need to do—weddings and funerals and building dedications, things like that. Whenever I counsel someone who feels called to be an evangelist, I always urge them to guard their time and not feel like they have to do everything. I also would have steered clear of politics. I'm grateful for the opportunities God gave me to minister to people in high places; people in power have spiritual and personal needs like everyone else, and often they have no one to talk to. But looking back I know I sometimes crossed the line, and I wouldn't do that now.[3]

Most would agree that Billy Graham's life was one of integrity, yet even he admitted he had regrets. In the same way, it is important for us to recognize our weak history markers so they can become directional arrows as we face future crossroads. While the past is behind us, our mistakes need not misdirect us for the rest of our lives. As people of integrity, we can be honest about our failures and misjudgments. We can allow them to be lessons that teach not only ourselves but also others within our personal sphere of influence.

Today, think about how a mistake you have made in regard to your personal health (whether physical, mental, emotional, or spiritual) could become a lesson you use to teach others in the future.

Lord, I am so thankful that You are a God of second chances. Thank You for extending grace to me so that I can turn the regrets of my life into lessons. In Jesus's name, amen

—— DAY 7: REFLECTION AND APPLICATION

Lord, it is difficult to lead a life of authenticity. Help me to always look to Jesus as my model for authentic living so I can reflect His example to the world. In Jesus' name, amen.

Archivists are people who assess whether a given piece of information—a document, letter, photograph, or recording—is of value and then maintain and store that information in an appropriate manner. They work to verify that something is authentic. For example, you might seek the services of an archivist if you wanted to document the authenticity of a family letter traced back to a famous person to determine its value (whether monetary or otherwise).

Archivists are also involved in acquiring important documents and preserving them. To this end, the Society of American Archivists has created some standards when it comes to verifying the authenticity of a document. We can learn much from these standards as we seek to become people of integrity:

> Authenticity is closely associated with the creator (or creators) of a record. First and foremost, an authentic record must have been created by the individual represented as the creator. The presence of a signature serves as a fundamental test for authenticity; the signature identifies the creator and establishes the relationship between the creator and the record.

> Authenticity can be verified by testing physical and formal characteristics of a record. The ink used to write a document must be contemporaneous with the document's purported date. The style and language of the document must be consistent with other related documents that are accepted as authentic.

> Authenticity alone does not automatically imply that the content of a record is reliable.[4]

As Christian people of integrity, we want to demonstrate authenticity in our likeness to our Creator. We want our record of authenticity to be the accumulation of the words we speak, the actions we demonstrate, and the attitudes we display through our demeanor. We want the signature of proof to be the Holy Spirit-breathed Word living in us and through us.

When we live with integrity, others will be able to verify our character through the everyday testing we face. We will respond with grace to cranky family members, refuse to lash out in the face of gossip or criticism, pursue godly courses of action when no one is watching, and have an inner attitude that reflects our values in Christ. The ink we will leave on others' lives is Light-written—completely traceable to the Sovereign One. Our style, language, smile, and lingering impressions will deeply pierce into the archives of others' thoughts and souls—and leave lasting, meaningful impressions that can transform them forever into eternity.

Read John 3:19-21. What has come into the world (see verse 19)? Fill in the blanks below.

"_____ has come into the _____, but _____ loved _____
instead of _____ because their _____ were _____."

The word *light* in this sentence comes from a Greek word that means "reaching the mind" or "evident." The word has been used to portray the Lord Jesus as the illuminator of men. Jesus becomes our illuminator—or "archivist authenticator"—when we compare our lives against His. Who loves the light, and who loves the darkness (see verses 20-21)?

_____

_____

_____

As as seekers of authenticity, we have the opportunity to make a difference on this earth by the way we live. Think about those people whom you hope will notice the imprint of Christ in your life. Pray today for any needs they may have and that they will see Jesus's integrity in you. Then pray that God will continue to mold and make you into His authentic document that testifies to His greatness.

Lord, I want to live out the authenticity of my faith by proclaiming the truth with both words and actions. Help me sincerely live out who I claim to be. In Jesus's name, amen!

1. Henry Schulman, "Why Affeldt Turned Down $500,000," *The San Francisco Chronicle*, May 15, 2013, accessed October 10, 2015, http://www.sfchronicle.com/giants/article Why-Affeldt-turned-down-500-000-4516372.php?t=34be181634999e0292.

2. John Ortberg, *Who Is This Man?* (Grand Rapids, MI: Zondervan, 2012), 49.

3. Sarah Pulliam Bailey, "Q&A: Billy Graham on Aging, Regrets, and Evangelicals," *Christianity Today*, January 21, 2001, accessed October 10, 2015, http://www.christianitytoday.com/ct/2011/januaryweb-only/qabillygraham.html?start=1.

4. "Authenticity," Society of American Archivists, accessed October 16, 2015, http://www2.archivists.org/glossary/terms/a/authenticity.

WEEK TEN: TRAINING IN HUMILITY

SCRIPTURE MEMORY VERSE
Be completely humble and gentle; be patient, bearing with one another in love.
Ephesians 4:2

Humble people are not out for any award. They have a modest view of themselves and posture themselves under others—not because they fail to recognize their contributions to society but because they value others more than themselves. One such person was Mother Teresa, a Catholic nun from Albania who founded the Missionaries of Charity in Calcutta, India. Her work was recognized by the world, and she received the Nobel Peace Prize in 1979.

The day after she received the award, she delivered a lecture in Norway in which she demonstrated her love for what Jesus termed the "least of these." She told a story of going out one evening to minister to people on the streets. One woman she met was in terrible condition, and she said to her fellow sisters, "You take care of the other three; I take care of this one." Mother Teresa put the woman in bed and did all she could do to help her. Sometime later, the woman, with a beautiful smile on her face, took hold of Mother Teresa's hand, said, "thank you," and then died. Mother Teresa said:

> I could not help but examine my conscience before her, and I asked what would I say if I was in her place. And my answer was very simple. I would have tried to draw a little attention to myself, I would have said I am hungry, that I am dying, I am cold, I am in pain, or something. But she gave me much more—she gave me her grateful love. And she died with a smile on her face. . . . This is the greatness of our people. And that is why we believe what Jesus had said: "I was hungry—I was naked—I was homeless—I was unwanted, unloved, uncared for—and you did it to me."[1]

This Nobel Peace Prize winner saw herself as less than a Calcutta homeless woman. This what it means to live out our Personal Trainer's characteristic of humility.

—— DAY 1: LIVE SIMPLY

Father, in a world caught up with accumulating material things, remind me that I live for You, for You value a focus on that which is eternal. In Jesus's name, amen.

Although we often seek blessings that come in the form of pay raises, vacations, and material objects like clothing, gifts, chocolate, or flowers, Jesus taught that blessings with eternal value come in other forms. Read Matthew 5:1-10. In this passage, the word translated blessed comes from a Greek word that means "length" in relationship to happiness. So, the blessedness or happiness Jesus speaks of here refers to a lasting state of joy—a feeling that is not fleeting and doesn't fade in the face of difficulty. In the following chart, write what you think Jesus meant by each term, and then write what blessing He said that person will receive.

Group of People	What This Means	How They Will Be Blessed
"the poor in spirit" (v. 3)		
"those who mourn" (v. 4)		
"the meek" (v. 5)		
"those who hunger and thirst for righteousness" (v. 6)		
"the merciful" (v. 7)		
"the pure in heart" (v. 8)		
"the peacemakers" (v. 9)		
"those who are persecuted because of righteousness" (v. 10)		

What is something these various kinds of people have in common?

_____
_____
_____

How could such people experience a long-term sense of happiness?

_____
_____
_____

Each group demonstrates a characteristic associated with those who are humble in nature. They live by their Christian faith, think less of themselves, suffer without complaint, demonstrate compassion for others in spite of their condition, and take on the role of peacemakers. Which group do you identify with the most? Why?

_____
_____
_____

Lord, make me Your humble instrument, attuned to the world around me and less concerned about myself. Be glorified in me, Lord. In Jesus's name, amen.

—— DAY 2: PUT OTHERS FIRST

Father, I truly want to develop a practice of serving others. Show me through Your Son's example of servanthood how to become humble in heart. In Jesus's name, amen.

Humble people don't rush to the front of the potluck line of life. They sit back, look out for others, and help them fill their plates. Though they may be leaders, they see themselves as servants of all. Our Personal Trainer emulated this lifestyle when He washed the disciples' feet at the Last Supper. Read John 13:1-17. What was Jesus's motivation for doing this (see verse 1)?

_____
_____
_____

In Jesus's day people traveled dusty roads, so they needed a sponge bath for their feet and hands when they arrived at a home—especially prior to a meal. A servant would typically perform this menial task. What was Jesus trying to teach the disciples?

How did Peter initially respond (see verses 6-8)? Why do you think he responded this way?

_____

_____

_____

What charge did Jesus give the disciples following this foot-washing (see verses 14-15)?

_____

_____

_____

What final lesson did Jesus teach about servanthood (see verse 16)?

_____

_____

_____

In verse 17, Jesus said that serving others will bless us. People often say they experience their greatest joy when they are helping others in need. Why does such a sense of blessing ensue from serving others?

_____

_____

_____

Take a moment to ask God to bring to mind someone you know who needs a servant leader's touch. How could you help him or her this week?

_____

_____

_____

Lord, Washer of Feet and Servant of All, I adore You. As I serve others, may I make a difference in the world so that others are drawn to You. In Jesus's name, amen.

—— DAY 3: SEEK TO SERVE

Father, I know all gifts come from You, so I need not boast about what I have done or who I am. Help me to use my gifts to lift up others and encourage them. In Jesus's name, amen.

Andrew Murray, a South African teacher and pastor, wrote, "The humble man feels no jealousy—or envy. He can praise God when others are preferred and blessed before him. He can bear to hear others praised and himself forgotten, because in God's presence he has learnt to say with Paul, 'I am nothing.' He has received the spirit of Jesus, who pleased not Himself, and sought not His own honor, as the spirit of his life."[2]

These traits make humble people great leaders. They appreciate strong relationships, are open to collaboration in the workplace and in ministry, and see the benefit of encouraging others to become their best. Humble people understand their strengths and weaknesses, know each person is valuable, and treat everyone with value. Jesus taught this principle of greatness to His disciples one time when He was asked a favor. Read Matthew 20:20-28. What did the mother of Jesus's disciples James and John ask Jesus (see verse 21)? What implication was behind the request?

_____

_____

_____

How did Jesus respond and what do you think he meant (see verses 22-23)?

_____

_____

_____

How did the other disciples feel about this request (see verse 24)? Why did they react this way?

_____

_____

_____

What did Jesus say was the difference between the way high officials acted as leaders and the new way He was teaching them (see verses 25-27)?

_____

_____

_____

How did Jesus fit this new model for servant leadership (see verse 28)?

_____

_____

_____

Think of a person you know who fits this definition of servant leader. What are some ways this person serves as a leader?

_____

_____

_____

Lord, thank You for teaching that true leadership is done by serving others. I will look for opportunities to help others because You gave Your life for many. In Jesus's name, amen.

—— DAY 4: HUMBLE YOURSELF

Father, You say that those who humble themselves will be viewed as the greatest in Your kingdom. Help me today to understand what it means to be humble. In Jesus's name, amen.

The word *humble* is not only an adjective but also a verb. We can humble ourselves by taking actions to become less arrogant, more modest, and less self-seeking in nature. Jesus taught this principle to His disciples. Read Matthew 18:1-4. What was the disciples' question (see verse 1)?

_____

_____

_____

In a parallel account given in Mark 9:33-37, we read the disciples had been arguing about this subject (see verse 34). Why would they be arguing?

_____

_____

_____

Whom does Jesus call over to serve as an example (see Matthew 18:2)?

_____

_____

_____

What action did Jesus say the disciples needed to take (see verse 3)?

_____

_____

_____

What are three effects of humbling yourself like a child (see Matthew 18:4 and Mark 9:37)?

_____

_____

_____

What does it mean to humble yourself like a child in terms of attitude and behavior?

_____

_____

_____

This week, think of one action you could take to humble yourself, such as picking up trash in your neighborhood, admitting you were wrong to a co-worker, or offering to serve in your church nursery. Commit to doing the task, but resist the urge to broadcast your good deed to others. Simply take joy in the fact that you have served "the least of these."

Lord, I take joy in the opportunity to welcome childlike humility into my heart—to rejoice in Your love, look for Your hand in my interactions, and trust You with sincere faith. In Jesus's name, amen.

—— DAY 5: BE THANKFUL

Father, on my own I am unworthy to untie Your Son's sandals. Therefore, I will continually bow my head in gratefulness for all You have given me through His sacrifice. In Jesus's name, amen.

In our quest to develop Christ-like qualities, having an attitude of gratitude will give us a right perspective of who we are in the greater picture of God's plan. Being thankful for what we have will make us appreciate God's provision, as opposed to having a sense that we have somehow earned what we have. Thankfulness softens the heart and makes us humble.

In *A Thankful Heart,* Carole Lewis, former First Place for Health national director, writes, "We can bring an attitude of thankfulness to any experience, and when we do, it's like a breath of fresh air rushing in and blowing away the dust of decay. . . . As we learn to cultivate a thankful heart, our grumbling and complaining will cease and be replaced by a spirit that blesses God, blesses those around us and even blesses ourselves. There is an answer to the question of what to do when life doesn't go perfectly: Give thanks in every situation in life."[3]

Gratitude can even be a form of worship. Read Luke 7:36-50. How did the woman express her gratitude to Jesus (see verses 37-38)?

_____

_____

_____

Why do you think she wanted to humbly serve Him this way?

_____

_____

_____

What was the Pharisee's objection (see verse 39)?

_____

_____

_____

How did Jesus explain His gratitude for her actions (see verses 44-47)?

_____

_____

_____

What gift did Jesus give to her (see verses 48-50)?

_____

_____

_____

A moment-by-moment awareness of God's provision will help us develop humility as we sense that each breath, opportunity, conversation, and new understanding provide ways to become closer to the Lord we love. For what are you thankful today?

_____

_____

_____

Carole Lewis wrote A Thankful Heart after her husband was diagnosed with stage IV cancer and her daughter was killed by a drunk driver. She found that thankfulness was part of the process of recovering from grief. For what difficult circumstances in your life could you give thanks?

_____

_____

_____

Consider sharing your decision to give thanks for something hard in your life with your group members to encourage them this week.

Lord, thank You for the blessings in my life and the hard circumstances too, as they are helping me develop humility as I learn to depend on You. In Jesus's name, amen.

—— DAY 6: REFLECTION AND APPLICATION

Father, You have given me so much, and I want to give back to others. Give me direction as to how to serve in my community, my church, and the world. In Jesus's name, amen.

Generosity is connected with humility. One very generous and humble man was Henry Crowell, the founder of the Quaker Oats Company, who reportedly knew how to use money carefully. When he began his business in a little Ohio factory, he promised God that he would honor Him in his giving. As Crowell realized God's favor was on him, he increased his giving until he was tithing 60 percent of his income, and continued doing so for more than 40 years. Crowell said, "I've never gotten ahead of God. He has always been ahead of me in giving."[4]

Giving helps us develop humility because it allows us to see how God can provide for us abundantly and be a part of His work on earth. Research shows that humble people tend to be more generous with their time and money, which is probably because their outlook is outward in nature and their time is more service-focused.[5] Humble people get caught up in projects that help individuals, their communities, and their churches, and worry less about themselves. They see life as God's journey and make connections to serve in a capacity that benefits others.

Our Personal Trainer expects us to give of our time, talents, and financial resources. The Bible shows He had a generous heart. There is no account of His refusing someone who asked for healing. He fed thousands who were hungry. He taught people to care for those in need regardless of who they were (see Luke 10:25-37). Because

God-in-the-Flesh was generous with His time, talents, and resources, He expects us to have a giving nature as well.

Generosity should be second nature to us, and we should give and serve without the expectation of applause. Jesus taught this concept to His disciples in Luke 17:7-10, where He gave an illustration of a servant who, after a day's work, then prepared a meal for his master. Jesus asked the disciples if the master would thank the servant for doing what he was told to do, and then said, "So you also, when you have done everything you were told to do, should say, 'We are unworthy servants; we have only done our duty'" (verse 10). When we are generous with our resources, that action in itself is our own reward.

How much should we give? Certainly, it's important to be prudent. After all, Jesus taught we should count the cost before starting a building project (see Luke 14:28-30). On the other hand, Jesus also taught that if someone forces us to go one mile, we should go an extra one (see Matthew 5:41). In the next breath He said, "Give to the one who asks you, and do not turn away from the one who wants to borrow from you" (Matthew 5:42). This week, consider how you might give of the gifts with which the Lord has blessed you.

Lord, serving in Your name is such a privilege! I see how being generous with my time and my financial resources can build my faith and make me more reliant on You. Thank You for teaching me to follow You humbly in all areas of my life. In Jesus's name, amen.

—— DAY 7: REFLECTION AND APPLICATION
Father, in a world caught up with accumulating material possessions, remind me that I live for You and that You value a focus on that which is eternal. In Jesus's name, amen.

If you learned today that in a matter of minutes Jesus was going to visit you in your home, how would you respond? Would you rush around and pick things up? Wash the car? Hide the unfolded laundry? Perhaps you would feel the same as one humble man in the Bible who did not feel worthy of having Jesus step across the threshold of his home.

When Jesus entered Capernaum, a city on the northwest side of the Sea of Galilee, several men asked Him to go to the home of a centurion, whose beloved servant was ill. Centurions were so named because they typically were in charge of a company of 100 Roman soldiers in Herod's army. This centurion sent Jewish elders to Jesus to come heal his servant. They begged Jesus, "This man deserves to have you do this, because he loves our nation and has built our synagogue" (Luke 7:4-5).

Jesus did go with them, but when He was close to the man's home, other friends of the centurion gave Jesus the man's message: "Lord, don't trouble yourself, for I do not deserve to have you come under my roof. That is why I did not even consider myself worthy to come to you. But say the word, and my servant will be healed. For I myself am a man under authority, with soldiers under me. I tell this one, 'Go,' and he goes; and that one, 'Come,' and he comes. I say to my servant, 'Do this,' and he does it" (Luke 7:6-8).

Jesus turned to the crowd that was following Him and said, "I tell you, I have not found such great faith even in Israel" (verse 9). When the men returned to the centurion's house, they found the servant healed. This story demonstrates the humility of this Roman officer—who certainly could have commanded Jesus to come. Yet he recognized the greater authority of Jesus, the Son of God, who could heal the sick without apparently even a word. The centurion's statement provides a few final points on humility:

1. **Humble people understand they do not deserve the grace of God**. The centurion said he was not worthy enough to welcome Christ into his own home. Feeling unworthy shows we understand our sinful condition as compared to the greatness of God.

2. **Humble people recognize faith is a gift of God.** The centurion demonstrated faith in Christ. A relationship with Christ is not something we can earn or something we deserve because of an accumulation of merits based on the good we have done. It is God's gift to us.

3. **Humble people recognize their own frailty.** The centurion recognized that Jesus could heal his servant with just a word—and that Christ did not even need to be in the presence of the sick man to do that healing. Even though the centurion had earthly command over 100 soldiers, his importance was worthless in terms of saving someone about whom he cared greatly. He had limited authority, whereas Jesus had authority over heaven and earth.

Running to Jesus with faith keeps arrogance at bay and gives God the opportunity to do His heaven work on earth—the healing of emotions, spirit, mind, and body. It helps us realize we cannot fix the problems of our loved ones and must rely completely on

Him for help. It also helps us recognize that Jesus's spirit indwells us and empowers us to be His hands and His feet on this earth. This was what Mother Teresa recognized in her life. When she gave her acceptance speech for the Nobel Peace Prize, she began with this prayer that Francis of Assisi popularized:

Lord, make a channel of Thy peace that, where there is hatred, I may bring love; that where there is wrong, I may bring the spirit of forgiveness; that, where there is discord, I may bring harmony; that, where there is error, I may bring truth; that, where there is doubt, I may bring faith; that, where there is despair, I may bring hope; that, where there are shadows, I may bring light; that, where there is sadness, I may bring joy. Lord, grant that I may seek rather to comfort than to be comforted, to understand than to be understood; to love than to be loved; for it is by forgetting self that one finds; it is forgiving that one is forgiven; it is by dying that one awakens to eternal life.[6]

As you seek to become more like your Personal Trainer, He will develop a humble heart within you. As you do, you will find your inspiration in the One who "being found in appearance as a man, he humbled himself by becoming obedient to death— even death on a cross! Therefore God exalted him to the highest place and gave him the name that is above every name, that at the name of Jesus every knee should bow . . . and every tongue confess that Jesus Christ is Lord, to the glory of God the Father" (Philippians 2:8-11).

Lord, bearing Your name is humbling, because I recognize that You gave everything for me and I have given so little back. Keep me mindful of Your great gift through Your Son, Jesus, that I may give others a glimpse of what it means to be Your follower. In Jesus's name, amen.

Notes

1. Mother Teresa, "Nobel Lecture," speech given December 11, 1979, accessed October 17, 2015, http://www.nobelprize.org/nobel_prizes/peace/laureates/1979/teresa-lecture.html.

2. Andrew Murray, *Humility* (New York: Anson D.F. Randolph & Co., 1895), cited on World Invisible, accessed October 17, 2005, http://www.worldinvisible.com/library/murray/5f00.0565/5f00.0565.06.htm.

3. Carole Lewis, *A Thankful Heart* (Ventura, CA: Regal, 2005), 14.

4. George Sweeting, "Money: Blessing or Curse?" *Moody*, April 1981, 1.

5. Michael W. Austin, "Humility Is a Trait Worth Having," *Psychology Today*, June 27, 2012, accessed October 17, 2015, https://www.psychologytoday.com/blog/ethics-everyone/201206/humility.

6. Mother Teresa, "Nobel Lecture."

WEEK ELEVEN: REVIEW AND REFLECT

To help you shape your short victory celebration testimony, work through the following questions in your prayer journal, one on each day leading up to your group's celebration:

DAY ONE: List some of the benefits you have gained by allowing the Lord to transform your life through this twelve-week First Place for Health session. Be mindful that He has been active in all four aspects of your being, so list benefits you have received in the physical, mental, emotional and spiritual realms.

DAY TWO: In what ways have you most significantly changed mentally? Have you seen a shift in the ways you think about yourself, food, your relationships, or God? How has Scripture memory been a part of these shifts?

DAY THREE: In what ways have you most significantly changed emotionally? Have you begun to identify how your feelings influence your relationship to food and exercise? What are you doing to stay aware of your emotions, both positive and negative?

DAY FOUR: In what ways have you most significantly changed spiritually? How has your relationship with God deepened? How has drawing closer to Him made a difference in the other three areas of your life?

DAY FIVE: In what ways have you most significantly changed physically? Have you met or exceeded your weight/measurement goals? How has your health improved during the past twelve weeks?

DAY SIX: Was there one person in your First Place for Health group who was particularly encouraging to you? How did their kindness make a difference in your First Place for Health journey?

DAY SEVEN: Summarize the previous six questions into a one-page testimony, or "faith story," to share at your group's victory celebration.

WEEK TWELVE: A TIME TO CELEBRATE!

Join your group in celebrating the benefits you have gained, the shift in the way you see yourself, how your relationship with God has changed, and the improvement in your health. Spend time celebrating your group and the encouragement you have experienced through each other. Celebrate!

LEADER DISCUSSION GUIDE

For in-depth information, guidance and helpful tips about leading a successful First Place for Health group, spend time studying the *My Place for Leadership* book. In it, you will find valuable answers to most of your questions, as well as personal insights from many First Place for Health group leaders.

For the group meetings in this session, be sure to read and consider each week's discussion topics several days before the meeting—some questions and activities require supplies and/or planning to complete. Also, if you are leading a large group, plan to break into smaller groups for discussion and then come together as a large group to share your answers and responses. Make sure to appoint a capable leader for each small group so that discussions stay focused and on track (and be sure each group records their answers!).

—— WEEK ONE: TRAINING IN DEVOTION

1. Ask if any of the members has had a personal trainer who helped them get more physically fit. Why would someone need a personal trainer? What strategies do personal trainers use to motivate their clients? How is Jesus like a personal trainer?
2. Ask someone to read the Lord's Prayer in Matthew 6:9-13. What are the different elements of the prayer? Why did Christ include them? Why should we keep our prayers simple?
3. Ask the group to share when and where they pray and study their Bible. Do they have a special quiet place to pray? Do they use a journal or list to record prayers and answers? Does anyone have creative ideas for someone who wanted to begin a quiet time? Jesus taught that our prayers should be simple—without lots of "babbling" (see Matthew 6:7). Ask the group if this is a surprising teaching—and why or why not.
4. Ask the group what they think of when they hear the word perseverance. Is this a quality they have? Why is it important to persist in our prayers?
5. Ask someone to read Jesus's teaching about boldness in Luke 11:5-13. How would they respond if a neighbor knocked on their door asking for food at midnight? Why is this example of boldness important as they approach God in prayer?
6. Explain that a mustard seed is the size of a dot that a fine-tipped pen would make. Jesus taught we only need faith the size of a mustard seed as we pray for

miracles. How big is their faith in comparison? The size of an almond? An apple? A watermelon? What amazing answers to prayer have they seen in their lives or the lives of those they know?

7. Ask the members to share one of their goals or dreams they will be praying for during the coming weeks. Close with prayer, thanking God for His desire to spend time with us and asking Him to make us more devoted through the practice of prayer and the study of His Word.

—— WEEK TWO: TRAINING IN FORGIVENESS

1. Ask someone to read the Lord's Prayer in Matthew 6:9-13. Ask which is harder: to forgive someone or to ask someone's forgiveness? Why?
2. State that Jesus taught we should forgive again and again. Obviously, in cases of abuse some kind of intervention should occur, but should there be limits on how we should forgive others? Why or why not?
3. This week the group read an amusing story about a little girl who sang, "Wet it go! Wet it go!" Explain that while it may be difficult to completely forget an offense, we can choose whether to remain judgmental and angry. Ask the group how they could "let it go" instead of holding on to a grudge.
4. In To Kill a Mockingbird Atticus Finch taught his children to put themselves in another person's shoes before judging them. What does it mean to put ourselves in someone else's shoes? How does that change our opinions about someone?
5. Ask the group how forgiveness could allow them to be healthier physically, mentally, emotionally, and spiritually.
6. Share about a time when you forgave yourself and ask the group if they can recall a similar time. Which is harder: to forgive someone else or to forgive ourselves? Why?
7. Close with prayer, thanking God for His grace and forgiveness for our past, present, and future sins. Ask Him to show the group how to keep their relationships clean with the practice of forgiveness.

—— WEEK THREE: TRAINING IN DETERMINATION

1. Explain that this week's lesson was about developing determination. Christ led a focused, purposeful, and determined life that revealed how to have a relationship with God. Ask the members if they have a sense of what their life's purpose is.

2. State that some people set priorities with to-do lists, while others live by calendars. How does the group generally set their priorities on a daily, weekly, or monthly basis?

3. Ask the group to recall the story of the preacher and the out-of-work man in Charles Sheldon's book In His Steps. How should the question "What Would Jesus Do?" influence their daily choices?

4. Ask the members to consider what situations in their lives cause them to draw on perseverance. How are they persevering with their First Place 4 Health goals?

5. Ask if there are any who would admit they are procrastinators. Did they relate to any of the reasons given this week for procrastination, including fear, perfectionism, avoidance of displeasure, or busyness? In what kinds of activities do they tend to procrastinate?

6. Explain that distractions keep us from achieving our goals. Ask the group what kinds of distractions are problematic for them—and if they have a solution for controlling them.

7. State that most people do not like criticism, but sometimes it can be helpful. Ask the members to recall a time when criticism brought about positive results.

8. Close in prayer, thanking God for giving our lives purpose and direction. Ask Him for clarity in helping the group live out that purpose on a daily basis.

—— WEEK FOUR: TRAINING IN RESOURCEFULNESS

1. Explain that resourceful people learn from the past. Ask one or two of the group members to share about something that taught them a lesson.

2. Ask a volunteer to read Romans 12:2. What would it take to transform a life—to break old habits and patterns and live anew?

3. State that people sometimes have a hard time delegating tasks, even when they are overwhelmed. Have the group members ever had a hard time delegating? What benefits did they receive when they did delegate?

4. Discuss why resourceful people are good time managers. Ask the members to suggest ways to use time more efficiently. What tips do they have to get work done?

5. Explain that Scripture is a tremendous resource when we need to solve problems, resist temptation, and seek guidance. Ask a volunteer to read about the temptation of Jesus in the desert in Matthew 4:1-11. How did Jesus use Scripture to resist temptation? What passages of Scripture are important to them? In what ways are those verses important?

6. Ask the group how spiritual disciplines such as praying and reading the Bible can help them be more resourceful physically, mentally, emotionally, and spiritually.

7. Close in prayer, thanking God for giving us His Word and the Holy Spirit to help us through the challenges of our lives. Ask God to continue developing the quality of resourcefulness in the members by helping them memorize and use Scripture.

—— WEEK FIVE: TRAINING IN WISDOM

1. Explain that our Personal Trainer, Jesus Christ, demonstrated great wisdom because He was not only human but also the Son of God. Ask the group whom they consider to be the wisest person in their lives—and how that person has influenced them.

2. State that mentors are those who nurture Christians in their faith and direct them as they face crossroads. Ask if anyone in the group has ever had a mentor. What was that experience like?

3. Recall how Henry Blackaby and Claude King taught in *Experiencing God* that Christians can know God's will through the Bible, prayer, other people, and experience. Ask the group how they best discern God's will for their lives.

4. Ask the members to explain how they make everyday decisions. Do they do research, go by instinct, or rely on some other way? How have they have learned from a mistake they made?

5. Ask someone to read Matthew 11:1-9. How did John the Baptist discern the truth about Jesus Christ? Discuss with the group how the characteristic of wisdom relates to their First Place for Health goals.

6. Explain that while some people learn through reading, others learns through experience. How is God nurturing the characteristic of wisdom in their lives through their study of Scripture or the experiences they have had?

7. Close in prayer, thanking God for creating us in His image and for giving us wisdom to guide our days. Ask God to increase the members' understanding by seeking wise counselors and spending time studying His Word.

—— WEEK SIX: TRAINING IN FAITHFULNESS

1. Explain that this week's study was about the faithfulness of Christ. Ask the group members how someone they know demonstrated the quality of faithfulness.

2. Ask a volunteer to read the story of Lazarus in John 11:1-44. How do the group members feel about Jesus's friendship toward Mary, Martha, and Lazarus?

3. Ask the group to define what principles a Christian should display in the work-place. How would someone demonstrate faithfulness to the organization? Should there be limits to that faithfulness?

4. Explain that faithfulness is a desired characteristic when serving in a ministry position. What would be the group's ideal kind of ministry—one they could see themselves sticking to for a long time?

5. Discuss how the Golden Rule has become a universal principle for how to treat others (see Luke 6:31). How does following this Jesus-taught principle help believers in Christ to remain faithful through conflicts? What does it mean to treat others as we would like to be treated? How would that look in practice?

6. Ask members how they typically spend the Sabbath (Sunday). Do they spend time in worship and rest? How could observing the Sabbath help develop the quality of faithfulness?

7. Close in prayer, thanking God for His faithfulness to us throughout the genera-tions—and especially through the example of His Son, Jesus Christ. Ask God to help the members be faithful in their relationships with family, friends, co-work-ers, neighbors, and ministry workers, and to be faithful representatives of Christ in times of conflict.

—— WEEK SEVEN: TRAINING IN COMPASSION

1. Ask a volunteer to read Jesus's teaching about the Greatest Commandment in Mark 12:28-34. Discuss how the second greatest commandment, "love your neighbor as yourself," might relate to the Greatest Commandment.

2. Explain that in a world where everyone is busy, it is challenging to be "in the moment"—to notice others around us. Ask the group how they notice the needs of people around them.

3. Remind the group that the Greek roots of the word empathy mean to be "in feel-ing" with someone else. Ask what kinds of situations cause their hearts to break.

4. Discuss how the members like to give encouragement to someone—such as through a text, an email, a little note in the mail, or a phone call. Ask them to remember times when someone's encouragement helped them through a tough time.

5. Recall the story of the man on the New York subway from Day Five. How did the story affect the group?

6. Ask the group to consider how loving the Lord with all their heart, soul, mind, and strength relates to their First Place for Health goals

7. Choose a volunteer to read Luke 19:41-44. Invite the group to consider how it would feel to see and hear Jesus sob over the city of Jerusalem—or over their own city.

8. Close in prayer, thanking God for demonstrating compassion by sending His Son, Jesus, for our sake. Ask God to make the group more loving with those around them so others see Christ at work in their lives.

—— WEEK EIGHT: TRAINING IN COMPOSURE

1. Explain that Jesus demonstrated composure in His dealings with those who were threatened by His ministry and the things He said and did. So, to be people of composure, we need to learn to abide in Christ. Ask someone to read the vine and branches teaching from John 15:1-17, and then discuss the connection between patience and abiding/remaining in Christ.

2. In Day Two the suggestion was made that a person can simply "refuse to be offended" when insults or criticism come. Ask the members how they tend to handle criticism or insults.

3. Ask a few volunteers to share about a time when they felt betrayed—and if that incident helped them identify with Christ.

4. Explain that John 17 is the chapter-long prayer Jesus prayed in the Upper Room before His arrest and crucifixion. Ask the group how the prayer helped them understand Jesus's love for others and His Father. How did prayer help Jesus have composure before going into the most difficult days of His life on earth?

5. Invite the group to share how fears can be destructive. How have they have learned to overcome fears and become more composed in difficult situations?

6. State there are things that trigger our emotional reactions—things that family members say, actions people do that bug us, traffic slowdowns, and more. Ask the group if there are particular triggers that cause unthinking emotional responses in them. How could they retrain their thinking so they respond with more composure?

7. Ask the group if they have someone they particularly admire who demonstrates composure under fire.

8. Close in prayer, thanking God for the many examples of how Christ demonstrated composure under persecution. Pray that God would help the group learn to be patiently positive in challenging situations by seeking His help and trusting Him for the results.

—— WEEK NINE: TRAINING IN INTEGRITY

1. Explain that this week's study was about the characteristic of integrity. Ask the group how the presence of the Holy Spirit in Christians' lives can help them live a life of integrity.
2. Ask the members how they are doing with their weekly Bible study. In what ways has it helped them meet their First Place 4 Health goals—physically, mentally, emotionally, and spiritually?
3. Discuss how Jesus valued people. How is His example a model for us as we try to live out our Christian faith? How is valuing people tied to the development of integrity?
4. Talk about what Jesus said about hypocrites—people whose walk does not match their talk—in Luke 6:37-42. Now ask the group if any of them have been inspired by another Christian in their faith walk. What was that person like?
5. Explain that pursuing excellence is essential for Christians so that others look to us as hard-working people of integrity. Choose someone to read Matthew 5:13-16. What is the function of salt? What is the function of light? What does it mean to be salt and light in the world?
6. Review Billy Graham's statement in Day Six about his regrets. Ask the group if they were surprised by any of his words.
7. Discuss what it means to be authentic in our faith. What struggles do the group members have in growing emotionally, spiritually, mentally, or physically?
8. Close in prayer, thanking God for sending Jesus Christ as the light of the world. Ask God to make the group "lamps" in their homes, neighborhoods, work places, and beyond.

—— WEEK TEN: TRAINING IN HUMILITY

1. Ask the group to define the word humility. What are some examples of how that characteristic might be demonstrated in people's lives?
2. Ask a volunteer to read the Beatitudes—often called the "be attitudes"—found in Mathew 5:1-10. Does anyone struggle with one or more of the "be attitudes"? What would be the hardest to live out?
3. Ask if any of the members have experienced a foot-washing ceremony. What did that signify for them? What could it signify in terms of developing humility on the part of the foot washer and the person whose feet were being washed?
4. Discuss what the members think of when they hear the term servant

leadership. How did Jesus model that form of leadership with His disciples and others?

5. Request a volunteer to read Matthew 18:1-4 and Luke 9:33-36. What kind of message was Jesus trying to deliver to His disciples who were jockeying for preference?

6. Ask the group what thankfulness has to do with the character quality of humility—and for what they are thankful personally.

7. Select a volunteer to read the prayer from St. Francis of Assisi in Day Seven. Ask the members what part of that prayer speaks to them about humility and the character of Christ.

8. Close in prayer, thanking God for sending His Son, Jesus, to earth to face rejection and humiliation for the sake of our salvation. Ask God to continue to show the group how to live a servant lifestyle so they can be Christ's hands and feet on this earth.

—— WEEK ELEVEN: REVIEW AND REFLECT

Be creative as you plan your Victory Celebration. Remember you're celebrating what God has accomplished during your groups 12-week session. Spend time celebrating your group and the encouragement you have experienced through each other. Give each member an opportunity to share their review and reflection. Celebrate the successes and milestones accomplished. See the "Planning a Victory Celebration" in *My Place for Leadership*.

—— WEEK ELEVEN: TIME TO CELEBRATE

FIRST PLACE FOR HEALTH
JUMP START MENUS

All recipe and menu nutritional information was determined using the Master-Cook software, a program that accesses a database containing more than 6,000 food items prepared using the United States Department of Agriculture (USDA) publications and information from food manufacturers. As with any nutritional program, MasterCook calculates the nutritional values of the recipes based on ingredients. Nutrition may vary due to how the food is prepared, where the food comes from, soil content, season, ripeness, processing and method of preparation. For these reasons, please use the recipes and menu plans as approximate guides. As always, consult your physician and/or a registered dietitian before starting a weight-loss program.

For those who need more calories,
add the following to the 1,400–1,500 calorie plan:

1,500-1,600 calories:	1 oz.-eq of protein, 1 oz.-eq. grains, ½ cup vegetables, 1 tsp. healthy oils
1,700-1,800 calories:	1½ oz.-eq. of protein, 2 oz.-eq. grains, 1 cup of vegetables, 1 tsp. healthy oils
1,900-2,000 calories:	2 oz.-eq. of protein, 2 oz.-eq. of grains, 1 cup vegetables, ½ cup fruit, 1 tsp. healthy oils
2,100-2,200 calories:	3 oz.-eq. of protein, 3 oz.-eq. grains, 1½ cup vegetables, ½ cup fruit, 2 tsp. healthy oils
2,300-2,400 calories:	4 oz.-eq. of protein, 4 oz.-eq. of grains, 2 cups vegetables 3 cups frit, 3 tsp. healthy oils

Raisin French Toast

1½ slices cinnamon-raisin bread
¼ cup egg substitute
¼ tsp. vanilla extract
1 tbsp. non-fat milk
nonstick cooking spray

In a shallow bowl, combine egg substitute, vanilla, and milk; add slices of bread, turning until egg mixture is absorbed. Spray a small nonstick skillet or griddle with nonstick cooking spray; preheat. Cook bread over medium heat 3 to 5 minutes, turning once, until golden brown on both sides. Serves 1.

Nutritional Information: 254 calories; 7g fat; 12g protein; 33g carbohydrate; 2g fiber; 1mg cholesterol; 278mg sodium

Fruity Chicken Salad

8 oz. chicken breast, cooked and diced
¼ cup celery, diced
1 apple, diced
½ cup seedless red grapes, halved
½ cup mandarin orange slices
2 walnut halves, chopped
1/3 cup low-fat mayonnaise
mixed lettuce leaves
4 tomatoes, quartered

Combine chicken, celery, apple, grapes, oranges, walnuts, and mayonnaise. Chill and serve on bed of lettuce with tomatoes as garnish. Serve with whole-grain crackers. Serves 4.

Nutritional Information: 376 calories; 24g fat; 22g protein; 22g carbohydrate; 5g fiber; 40mg cholesterol; 149mg sodium

BBQ Beef and Noodles

1 lb. lean ground beef
4 oz. egg noodles, uncooked
¾ cup water
2 tbsp. light margarine
¾ cup onion, diced
1 lb. mushrooms, sliced
2 egg yolks
3 tbsp. BBQ sauce
2 tbsp. cooking sherry

Bring water to a boil. Place noodles in heat-resistant mixing bowl; cover with boiling water. Set aside for 20 minutes; then drain. In nonstick skillet, melt margarine over medium heat. Add onion; sauté 5 minutes or until soft. Add beef and mushrooms to skillet; increase heat to high and cook for 5 additional minutes, stirring constantly. Add water; reduce heat to low and continue cooking another 10 minutes. While meat is cooking, mix together egg yolks, BBQ sauce, and sherry. Scoop several spoonfuls of the meat mixture into bowl of egg mixture. Turn contents of bowl into skillet; heat gently while stirring. Serve over noodles. Serves 4.

Nutritional Information: 450 calories; 30g fat; 26g protein; 17g carbohydrate; 2g fiber; 201mg cholesterol; 255mg sodium

Light and Fluffy Blueberry Pancakes

3 eggs
1 cup plain non-fat yogurt
¼ cup applesauce, unsweetened
½ tsp. vanilla extract
2 tbsp. sugar
1 tsp. baking soda
¼ tsp. salt
1 cup all-purpose flour
1 cup blueberries
nonstick cooking spray

Separate 1 egg white and yolk into 2 large bowls. Add whites only from remaining 2 eggs into egg-white bowl; save extra yolks in refrigerator. Add yogurt, applesauce, vanilla, and sugar to egg-yolk bowl; stir with rubber spatula to mix. Stir in baking soda, salt, and flour; blend well. Beat egg whites with electric mixer until stiff peaks form when beaters are lifted. Stir 1/3 of whites into batter until blended; gently fold in remaining whites until no white streaks remain. Preheat large skillet over medium heat until a few drops of water flicked onto the surface skitter around and then disappear. Coat griddle with nonstick cooking spray. Pour ¼ cup batter onto griddle; gently spreading to make a 4-inch pancake. If using fruit, quickly sprinkle on top; cook 2 minutes more or until bubbles appear on surface of pancake and underside is golden brown. Turn pancake over with broad metal spatula; cook 2 more minutes or until tops bounce back when touched. Makes 4 servings of 3 pancakes or 6 servings of 2 pancakes.

Nutritional Information: 236 calories; 5g fat; 11g protein; 35g carbohydrate; 2g fiber; 163mg cholesterol; 546mg sodium

Zucchini Salad

2 zucchini, peeled into ribbons
2 Roma tomatoes, diced
½ bell pepper, diced
¼ cup olives, chopped
¼ cup pine nuts
1 tbsp. fresh basil, chopped
1 small clove garlic, crushed
1-2 tbsp. extra-virgin olive oil
salt
black pepper
fresh lemon juice

Toss all ingredients in a bowl, adding salt, pepper, and lemon juice to taste. Serves 2.

Nutritional Information: 243 calories; 18g fat; 8g protein; 17g carbohydrate; 6g fiber; 0mg cholesterol; 192mg sodium

Salsa Meat Loaf

1 lb. lean ground beef
1 egg
2 tbsp. green bell pepper, finely chopped
1/3 cup onion, finely chopped
1 tsp. salt
2 slices bread, finely cubed
½ tsp. dry mustard
1/3 cup salsa

Preheat oven to 400° F. In a large bowl, combine all ingredients; mix well to form a loaf. Place loaf in foil-lined 5 x 9-inch baking pan; bake 40 to 45 minutes or until done. Serves 4.

Nutritional Information: 365 calories; 25g fat; 23g protein; 9g carbohydrate; 1g fiber; 138mg cholesterol; 790mg sodium

Open-Faced Hawaiian Breakfast Sandwich

1 English muffin, split
2 slices tomato
¾ oz. fat-free ham, sliced, cut in half
2 slices pineapple
1 slice low-fat cheese, cut in half

Top muffin halves with one slice each of tomato, ham, pineapple, and cheese. Place in hot oven until cheese is melted.

Nutritional Information: 270 calories; 5g fat; 18g protein; 40g carbohydrate; 4g fiber; 16mg cholesterol; 764mg sodium

Herbed Cheese and Tomato Sandwich

1 English muffin
¼ cup low-fat cottage cheese
2 slices tomato
¼ avocado
1 tbsp. spicy brown mustard
1 leaf green lettuce
1 tbsp. chives
garlic powder, to taste

Layer ingredients and enjoy.

Nutritional Information: 387 calories; 12g fat; 21g protein; 55g carbohydrate; 13g fiber; 2mg cholesterol; 774mg sodium

DAY 3 | DINNER

Texas Round Steak

1½ lbs. beef round steak, cut into 6 pieces
½ cup all-purpose flour
1 tsp. salt
2½ tsp. chili powder
1 tbsp. vegetable oil
½ cup green bell pepper, chopped
½ cup onion, chopped
1 cup fat-free beef broth
½ cup tomato juice
¼ tsp. garlic powder
¼ tsp. cumin

In shallow dish, blend flour, salt, and 1½ tsp. chili powder. Dredge meat in flour mixture (use about half of the mixture). Place oil in heavy skillet; heat to frying temperature over moderate heat. Add meat; brown on both sides. Transfer steaks to 1½-quart casserole dish; set aside. Use skillet to sauté pepper and onion, stirring frequently; remove with slotted spoon and spread over meat. Drain remaining fat from skillet; add beef broth. Cook over moderate heat to loosen brown particles remaining in skillet. Add tomato juice, remaining 1 tsp. chili powder, garlic powder, and cumin; mix well and pour over meat. Use fork to lightly distribute broth and vegetables over meat. Cover tightly; bake at 325❓ F for 1 to 1½ hours or until meat is tender. Top each serving of steak with sauce. Serves 6.

Nutritional Information: 293 calories; 16g fat; 25g protein; 12g carbohydrate; 1g fiber; 67mg cholesterol; 581mg sodium

Cantaloupe-Banana Smoothieza

1 cup vanilla-flavored non-fat yogurt
½ cantaloupe, peeled and cubed
1 banana, peeled and sliced

Combine all ingredients in a blender and purée until smooth. Serves 2.

Nutritional Information: 166 calories; 1g fat; 8g protein; 34g carbohydrate; 3g fiber; 2mg cholesterol; 100mg sodium

Garden Salad with Citrus Vinaigrette

Vinaigrette:
3 tbsp. orange juice
1½ tbsp. lime juice
2½ tsp. extra-virgin olive oil
2 tsp. honey
1 tsp. red wine vinegar
¼ tsp. salt
1/8 tsp. ground black pepper

Salad:
1½ cups (1 x ¼-inch) julienne-cut zucchini
1½ cups (1 x ¼-inch) julienne-cut yellow squash
1 cup corn kernels (about 2 ears)
2 tbsp. red onion, finely chopped
1 tbsp. fresh parsley, finely chopped
1 tbsp. fresh basil, finely chopped

To prepare vinaigrette, combine ingredients and stir with a whisk. To prepare salad, combine zucchini and remaining ingredients in a large bowl. Add vinaigrette; toss well. Cover and chill. Serves 4.

Nutritional Information: 96 calories; 3g fat; 2g protein; 17g carbohydrate; 3g fiber; 0mg cholesterol; 139mg sodium

Beef Stir-Fry

1 lb. lean beef sirloin
2 tsp. canola oil
1 tsp. garlic, chopped
4 oz. linguine noodles, uncooked
1 red onion, sliced
1 cup carrots, sliced
1 cup zucchini, diced
3 tbsp. water
1 cup fresh broccoli florets
1 cup mushrooms, sliced
1 tsp. soy sauce
nonstick cooking spray

Heat oil over high heat in skillet sprayed with nonstick cooking spray. Add beef and garlic; stir-fry until cooked to your liking. Remove from skillet; keep warm. Cook noodles according to package directions, omitting salt and fat. Drain and keep warm. Stir-fry onion and carrots until carrots are partially done, adding water as needed to prevent sticking. Add zucchini, broccoli, mushrooms, and soy sauce. (Note: Any combination of vegetables may be used.) Stir-fry until vegetables are done to your liking. Add beef to reheat; then toss with pasta. Serves 4.

Nutritional Information: 403 calories; 19g fat; 26g protein; 31g carbohydrate; 3g fiber; 72mg cholesterol; 164mg sodium

Power Breakfast Smoothie

¾ cup non-fat plain yogurt
1 cup orange juice
¾ cup apple, peeled and diced
1 banana, frozen
1 tsp. vanilla extract
3 tbsp. peanut butter
2 tbsp. wheat germ

Combine all ingredients in a blender and purée until smooth. Serves 4.

Nutritional Information: 179 calories; 7g fat; 7g protein; 24g carbohydrate; 3g fiber; 1mg cholesterol; 90mg sodium

DAY 5 | LUNCH

Apple Chicken Salad

2 boneless, skinless chicken breasts (pounded to half-inch thickness)
1 tsp. seasoning salt
6-8 cups mixed greens
2 medium tomatoes, cut into wedges
¼ red onion, thinly sliced
¾ cup pecan halves
½ cup feta cheese, crumbled
2 cups apple chips
1 cup Fuji apple salad dressing
Dressing:
2 tbsp. extra-virgin olive oil
1 tbsp. white balsamic vinegar
1 tbsp. apple cider vinegar
1 tbsp. garlic powder
1 tbsp. onion powder
1½ tsp. Dijon mustard
3 tbsp. frozen apple juice concentrate

Season chicken breasts with seasoning salt and cook on both sides for 3 to 4 minutes each in a greased skillet or pan over medium heat. Cut into pieces and set aside. In a large bowl, toss together mixed greens, tomatoes, sliced onions, and chicken. Sprinkle pecans, cheese crumbles, and apple chips on top. In separate bowl, whisk dressing ingredients. Serve with fuji apple dressing. Serves 4.

Nutritional Information: 311 calories; 18g fat; 24g protein; 13g carbohydrate; 3g fiber; 71mg cholesterol; 93mg sodium

Beef Kabobs

1 lb. lean sirloin, cut into 16 cubes
1 zucchini, sliced into rounds
1 red onion, quartered to make 12 pieces
1 green bell pepper, cut into 12 pieces
8 mushroom caps
2 tsp. extra-virgin olive oil
2 tsp. Worcestershire sauce
½ tsp. fresh oregano
¼ tsp. ground black pepper
12 cherry tomatoes

Skewer meat and vegetables in the following order: mushroom, meat cube, onion, zucchini, bell pepper, meat, onion, zucchini, bell pepper, meat, onion, zucchini, bell pepper, meat, and mushroom. Place kabobs in 13 x 9-inch glass dish; set aside. In small bowl, combine oil, Worcestershire sauce, oregano, and pepper; mix well and pour over kabobs. Cover dish and refrigerate overnight. Grill to desired doneness and garnish each with 3 cherry tomatoes. Serves 4.

Nutritional Information: 210 calories; 4g fat; 26g protein; 15g carbohydrate; 98mg cholesterol; 855mg sodium

DAY 6 | BREAKFAST

Almond Power Bar

1 cup old-fashioned rolled oats
¼ cup almonds, slivered
¼ cup sunflower seeds
1 tbsp. flaxseeds
1 tbsp. sesame seeds
1 cup unsweetened whole-grain puffed cereal
1/3 cup dried apricots, chopped
1/3 cup chopped golden raisins
¼ cup almond butter
¼ cup sugar
¼ cup honey
½ tsp. vanilla extract
1/8 tsp. salt
nonstick cooking spray

Preheat oven to 350° F. Coat an 8-inch square pan with nonstick cooking spray. Spread oats, almonds, sunflower seeds, flaxseeds, and sesame seeds on a large, rimmed baking sheet. Bake until the oats are lightly toasted and the nuts are fragrant, shaking the pan halfway through (about 10 minutes). Transfer to a large bowl. Add cereal, apricots, and raisins; toss to combine. Combine almond butter, sugar, honey, vanilla, and salt in a small saucepan. Heat over medium-low heat, stirring frequently, until the mixture bubbles lightly (2 to 5 minutes). Immediately pour the almond butter mixture over the dry ingredients and mix with a spoon or spatula until no dry spots remain. Transfer to the prepared pan. Lightly coat your hands with nonstick cooking spray and press the mixture down firmly to make an even layer (wait until the mixture cools slightly if necessary). Refrigerate until firm (about 30 minutes); cut into 8 bars. (Note: You can store in an airtight container at room temperature or in the refrigerator for up to 1 week or freeze for up to 1 month; thaw at room temperature.) Serves 8.

Nutritional Information: 244 calories; 10g fat; 5g protein; 38g carbohydrates; 3g fiber; 0mg cholesterol; 74mg sodium

Veggie Quinoa Salad

1 cup quinoa, rinsed
2 cups water
¼ tsp. salt
1½ cups frozen edamame, shelled
3 carrots, peeled and diced
½ yellow pepper, diced
½ red pepper, diced
1 cup red cabbage, chopped
2 tbsp. sesame oil
2 tbsp. rice vinegar
3 tsp. fresh ginger, finely minced
1 tbsp. sesame seeds

Place the quinoa, water, and salt in a covered pot. Heat on high until it boils, lower the heat to low, and cook for about 15 minutes or until the quinoa is soft and the water absorbed. Pour the quinoa into a medium-sized bowl and mix in the frozen edamame, carrots, peppers, and cabbage. In a small bowl, make the dressing by mixing the sesame oil, rice vinegar, minced ginger, and sesame seeds. Pour the dressing over the quinoa and veggies and mix thoroughly. Enjoy immediately, or store in a covered container for later. Serves 4.

Nutritional Information: 294 calories; 11g fat; 9g protein; 43g carbohydrate; 7g fiber; 0mg cholesterol; 170mg sodium

Pasta Primavera with Meat Sauce

1 lb. lean ground beef
6 oz. penne pasta, uncooked
¼ cup onion, diced
¼ cup red or green bell pepper, diced
1 cup mushrooms, sliced
1 tsp. granulated garlic
1 tsp. salt
3 cup spaghetti sauce
1 (10-oz.) pkg. frozen stir-fry vegetables, thawed
nonstick cooking spray

Cook pasta according to package directions, omitting salt and fat. Drain and set aside. In large saucepan coated with nonstick cooking spray, sauté onion and bell pepper. Add mushrooms, garlic, salt, and ground beef; cook 12 minutes or until done. Drain off excess fat; add spaghetti sauce and vegetables. Simmer for 5 minutes more; serve over pasta. Serves 4.

Nutritional Information: 551 calories; 24g fat; 30g protein; 51g carbohydrate; 5g fiber; 78mg cholesterol; 1388mg sodium

Chocolate Banana Oatmeal

1 cup water
pinch of salt
½ cup old-fashioned rolled oats (or 1/3 cup steel-cut oats)
½ banana, sliced
1 tbsp. chocolate-hazelnut spread
pinch of flaky sea salt

Bring water and a pinch of regular salt to a boil in a small saucepan. Stir in rolled oats, reduce heat to medium and cook, stirring occasionally, until most of the liquid is absorbed (about 5 minutes). Remove from heat, cover, and let stand 2 to 3 minutes. (Note: If using steel-cut oats, bring 1 cup water and a pinch of salt to a boil in a small saucepan. Add 1/3 cup steel-cut oats, reduce heat to a bare simmer, cover and cook, stirring occasionally, until most of the liquid is absorbed, 15 to 20 minutes. Remove from heat and let stand, covered, 2 to 3 minutes.) Top with banana, chocolate spread, and flaky salt. Serves 1.

Nutritional Information: 290 calories; 7g fat; 8g protein; 50g carbohydrate; 6g fiber; 0mg cholesterol; 275mg sodium

Southwestern Three-Bean Chili

1 tbsp. vegetable oil
1 lb. carrots
2 stalks celery
2 clove garlic
1 jumbo onion
4 tsp. chili powder
1 tbsp. cumin
½ tsp. cinnamon
¼ tsp. ground red pepper (cayenne)
1 tsp. salt
1 can tomatoes, diced
1 can vegetable broth
1 cup water
2 can white kidney beans (cannellini)
1 can pink beans
2 cup frozen edamame, shelled
¼ cup fresh cilantro leaves
reduced-fat sour cream (optional)
reduced-fat cheddar cheese, shredded (optional)

In 5- to 6-quart Dutch oven, heat vegetable oil on medium-high until hot. Add carrots, celery, garlic, and onion. Cook 10 to 12 minutes or until all vegetables are browned and tender, stirring occasionally. Stir in chili powder, cumin, cinnamon, ground red pepper, and salt; cook 30 seconds, stirring. Add tomatoes, broth, and water; heat to boiling. Reduce heat to low; cover and simmer 15 minutes. Stir white kidney beans and pink beans into Dutch oven; cover and cook 10 minutes longer. Stir in frozen edamame and cook, uncovered, 5 to 7 minutes or until edamame are just tender, stirring occasionally. Stir ¼ cup cilantro into chili. Spoon half of chili into serving bowls; garnish with cilantro leaves. Serve with sour cream and cheddar (if desired). Spoon remaining chili into freezer-safe containers. Serves 8.

Nutrition Information: 306 calories; 7g fat; 19g protein; 45g carbohydrate; 13g fiber; 0mg cholesterol; 521mg sodium

Mexican-Style Beef and Pasta

1 lb. (1-inch thick) round-tip steak, cut into ¼-inch thick strips
1 (4-oz.) pkg. rotini pasta, uncooked
1 tbsp. extra virgin olive oil
1 pkg. taco seasoning mix
1 tbsp. fresh cilantro, chopped
3 garlic cloves, crushed
2 cup chunky salsa (any kind)
1 (15-oz.) can black beans, rinsed and drained
½ cup water

Cook pasta according to package directions, omitting salt and fat. Drain and set aside. Combine steak strips, taco seasoning, cilantro, and garlic; toss to coat. Heat oil in skillet; sauté half of steak strips over high heat 1 to 2 minutes or until no longer pink. Remove with slotted spoon and repeat with remaining strips, removing all cooked strips from skillet. Add pasta, salsa, beans, and water to skillet; cook 4 to 5 minutes over medium heat. Combine with steak in serving bowl; garnish as desired. Serves 4.

Nutritional Information: 555 calories; 18g fat; 37g protein; 60g carbohydrate; 11g fiber; 67mg cholesterol; 1206mg sodium

STEPS FOR SPIRITUAL GROWTH

—— **GOD'S WORD FOR YOUR LIFE**

I have hidden your word in my heart that I might not sin against you. Psalm 119:11

As you begin to make decisions based on what God's Word teaches you, you will want to memorize what He has promised to those who trust and follow Him. Second Peter 1:3 tells us that God "has given us everything we need for life and godliness through our knowledge of him" (emphasis added). The Bible provides instruction and encouragement for any area of life in which you may be struggling. If you are dealing with a particular emotion or traumatic life event—fear, discouragement, stress, financial upset, the death of a loved one, a relationship difficulty—you can search through a Bible concordance for Scripture passages that deal with that particular situation. Scripture provides great comfort to those who memorize it.

One of the promises of knowing and obeying God's Word is that it gives you wisdom, insight, and understanding above all worldly knowledge (see Psalm 119:97–104). Psalm 119:129–130 says, "Your statutes are wonderful; therefore I obey them. The unfolding of your words gives light; it gives understanding to the simple." Now that's a precious promise about guidance for life!

The Value of Scripture Memory

Scripture memory is an important part of the Christian life. There are four key reasons to memorize Scripture:

> **TO HANDLE DIFFICULT SITUATIONS.** A heartfelt knowledge of God's Word will equip you to handle any situation that you might face. Declaring such truth as, "I can do everything through Christ" (see Philippians 4:13) and "he will never leave me or forsake me" (see Hebrews 13:5) will enable you to walk through situations with peace and courage.

> **TO OVERCOME TEMPTATION.** Luke 4:1–13 describes how Jesus used Scripture to overcome His temptations in the desert (see also Matthew 4:1-11). Knowledge of Scripture and the strength that comes with the ability to use it are important parts of putting on the full armor of God in preparation for spiritual warfare (see Ephesians 6:10–18).

TO GET GUIDANCE. Psalm 119:105 states the Word of God "is a lamp to my feet and a light for my path." You learn to hide God's Word in your heart so His light will direct your decisions and actions throughout your day.

TO TRANSFORM YOUR MIND. "Do not conform any longer to the pattern of this world, but be transformed by the renewing of your mind" (Romans 12:2). Scripture memory allows you to replace a lie with the truth of God's Word. When Scripture becomes firmly settled in your memory, not only will your thoughts connect with God's thoughts, but you will also be able to honor God with small everyday decisions as well as big life-impacting ones. Scripture memorization is the key to making a permanent lifestyle change in your thought patterns, which brings balance to every other area of your life.

Scripture Memory Tips

- Write the verse down, saying it aloud as you write it.
- Read verses before and after the memory verse to get its context.
- Read the verse several times, emphasizing a different word each time.
- Connect the Scripture reference to the first few words.
- Locate patterns, phrases, or keywords.
- Apply the Scripture to circumstances you are now experiencing.
- Pray the verse, making it personal to your life and inserting your name as the recipient of the promise or teaching. (Try that with 1 Corinthians 10:13, inserting "me" and "I" for "you.")
- Review the verse every day until it becomes second nature to think those words whenever your circumstances match its message. The Holy Spirit will bring the verse to mind when you need it most if you decide to plant it in your memory.

Scripture Memorization Made Easy!

What is your learning style? Do you learn by hearing, by sight, or by doing? If you learn by hearing—if you are an auditory learner—singing the Scripture memory verses, reading them aloud, or recording them and listening to your recording will be very helpful in the memorization process. If you are a visual learner, writing the verses and repeatedly reading through them will cement them in your mind.

If you learn by doing—if you are a tactile learner—creating motions for the words or using sign language will enable you to more easily recall the verse. After determining your learning style, link your Scripture memory with a daily task, such as driving to work, walking on a treadmill, or eating lunch. Use these daily tasks as opportunities to memorize and review your verses.

Meals at home or out with friends can be used as a time to share the verse you are memorizing with those at your table. You could close your personal email messages by typing in your weekly memory verse. Or why not say your memory verse every time you brush your teeth or put on your shoes?

The purpose of Scripture memorization is to be able to apply God's words to your life. If you memorize Scripture using methods that connect with your particular learning style, you will find it easier to hide God's Word in your heart.

—— ESTABLISHING A QUIET TIME

Like all other components of the First Place for Health program, developing a live relationship with God is not a random act. You must intentionally seek God if you are to find Him! It's not that God plays hide-and-seek with you. He is always available to you. He invites you to come boldly into His presence. He reveals Himself to you in the pages of the Bible. And once you decide to earnestly seek Him, you are sure to find Him! When you delight in Him, your gracious God will give you the desires of your heart. Spending time getting to know God involves four basic elements: a priority, a plan, a place, and practice.

A Priority

You can successfully establish a quiet time with God by making this meeting a daily priority. This may require carving out time in your day so you have time and space for this new relationship you are cultivating. Often this will mean eliminating less important things so you will have time and space to meet with God. When speaking about Jesus, John the Baptist said, "He must become greater; I must become less" (John 3:30). You will undoubtedly find that to be true as well. What might you need to eliminate from your current schedule so that spending quality time with God can become a priority?

A Plan

Having made quiet time a priority, you will want to come up with a plan. This plan will include the time you have set aside to spend with God and a general outline of how you will spend your time in God's presence.

Elements you should consider incorporating into your quiet time include:

- Singing a song of praise
- Reading a daily selection in a devotional book or reading a psalm
- Using a systematic Scripture reading plan so you will be exposed to the whole truth of God's Word
- Completing your First Place for Health Bible study for that day
- Praying—silent, spoken, and written prayer
- Writing in your spiritual journal.

You will also want to make a list of the materials you will need to make your encounter with God more meaningful:

- A Bible
- Your First Place for Health Bible study
- Your prayer journal
- A pen and/or pencil
- A devotional book
- A Bible concordance
- A college-level dictionary
- A box of tissues (tears—both of sadness and joy—are often part of our quiet time with God!)

Think of how you would plan an important business meeting or social event, and then transfer that knowledge to your meeting time with God.

A Place

Having formulated a meeting-with-God plan, you will next need to create a meeting-with-God place. Of course, God is always with you; however, in order to have quality devotional time with Him, it is desirable that you find a comfortable meeting place. You will want to select a spot that is quiet and as distraction-free as possible.

Meeting with God in the same place on a regular basis will help you remember what you are there for: to have an encounter with the true and living God!

Having selected the place, put the materials you have determined to use in your quiet time into a basket or on a nearby table or shelf. Now take the time to establish your personal quiet time with God. Tailor your quiet time to fit your needs—and the time you have allotted to spend with God. Although many people elect to meet with God early in the morning, for others afternoon or evening is best. There is no hard-and-fast rule about when your quiet time should be—the only essential thing is that you establish a quiet time!

Start with a small amount of time that you know you can devote yourself to daily. You can be confident that as you consistently spend time with God each day, the amount of time you can spend will increase as you are ready for the next level of your walk with God.

I will meet with God from _____ to _____ daily.

I plan to use that time with God to _____

_____

Supplies I will need to assemble include _____

_____

My meeting place with God will be _____

_____

Practice

After you have chosen the time and place to meet God each day and you have assembled your supplies, there are four easy steps for having a fruitful and worshipful time with the Lord.

STEP 1: Clear Your Heart and Mind

"Be still, and know that I am God" (Psalm 46:10). Begin your quiet time by reading the daily Bible selection from a devotional guide or a psalm. If you are new in your Christian walk, an excellent devotional guide to use is *Streams in the Desert* by L.B. Cowman. More mature Christians might benefit from *My Utmost for His Highest* by Oswald Chambers. Of course, you can use any devotional that has a strong emphasis on Scripture and prayer.

STEP 2: Read and Interact with Scripture

"I have hidden your word in my heart that I might not sin against you" (Psalm 119:11). As you open your Bible, ask the Holy Spirit to reveal something He knows you need for this day through the reading of His Word. Always try to find a nugget to encourage or direct you through the day. As you read the passage, pay special attention to the words and phrases the Holy Spirit brings to your attention. Some words may seem to resonate in your soul. You will want to spend time meditating on the passage, asking God what lesson He is teaching you.

After reading the Scripture passage over several times, ask yourself the following questions:

- In light of what I have read today, is there something I must now do? (Confess a sin? Claim a promise? Follow an example? Obey a command? Avoid a situation?)
- How should I respond to what I've read today?

STEP 3: Pray

"Be clear minded and self-controlled so that you can pray" (1 Peter 4:7). Spend time conversing with the Lord in prayer. Prayer is such an important part of First Place for Health that there is an entire section in this member's guide devoted to the practice of prayer.

STEP 4: Praise

"Praise the LORD, O my soul, and forget not all his benefits" (Psalm 103:2). End your quiet time with a time of praise. Be sure to thank the Lord of heaven and warmth for choosing to spend time with you!

—— SHARING YOUR FAITH

Nothing is more effective in drawing someone to Jesus than sharing personal life experiences. People are more open to the good news of Jesus Christ when they see faith in action. Personal faith stories are simple and effective ways to share what Christ is doing in your life, because they show firsthand how Christ makes a difference.

Sharing your faith story has an added benefit: it builds you up in your faith, too! Is your experience in First Place for Health providing you opportunities to share with others what God is doing in your life? If you answered yes, then you have a personal faith story! If you do not have a personal faith story, perhaps it is because you don't know Jesus Christ as your personal Lord and Savior. Read through "Steps to Becoming a Christian" (which is the next chapter) and begin today to give Christ first place in your life.

Creativity and preparation in using opportunities to share a word or story about Jesus is an important part of the Christian life. Is Jesus helping you in a special way? Are you achieving a level of success or peace that you haven't experienced in other attempts to lose weight, exercise regularly, or eat healthier? As people see you making changes and achieving success, they may ask you how you are doing it. How will—or do—you respond? Remember, your story is unique, and it may allow others to see what Christ is doing in your life. It may also help to bring Christ into the life of another person.

Personal Statements of Faith

First Place for Health gives you a great opportunity to communicate your faith and express what God is doing in your life. Be ready to use your own personal statement of faith whenever the opportunity presents itself. Personal statements of faith should be short and fit naturally into a conversation. They don't require or expect any action or response from the listener. The goal is not to get another person to change but simply to help you communicate who you are and what's important to you.

Here are some examples of short statements of faith that you might use when someone asks what you are doing to lose weight:

- "I've been meeting with a group at my church. We pray together, support each other, learn about nutrition, and study the Bible."

- "It's amazing how Bible study and prayer are helping me lose weight and eat healthier."
- "I've had a lot of support from a group I meet with at church."
- "I'm relying more on God to help me make changes in my lifestyle."

Begin keeping a list of your meaningful experiences as you go through the First Place for Health program. Also notice what is happening in the lives of others. Use the following questions to help you prepare short personal statements and stories of faith:

- What is God doing in your life physically, mentally, emotionally, and spiritually?
- How has your relationship with God changed? Is it more intimate or personal?
- How is prayer, Bible study, and/or the support of others helping you achieve your goals for a healthy weight and good nutrition?

Writing Your Personal Faith Story

Write a brief story about how God is working in your life through First Place for Health. Use your story to help you share with others what's happening in your life.

Use the following questions to help develop your story:

- Why did you join First Place for Health? What specific circumstances led you to a Christ-centered health and weight-loss program? What were you feeling when you joined?
- What was your relationship with Christ when you started First Place for Health? What is it now?
- Has your experience in First Place for Health changed your relationship with Christ? With yourself? With others?
- How has your relationship with Christ, prayer, Bible study, and group support made a difference in your life?
- What specific verse or passage of Scripture has made a difference in the way you view yourself or your relationship with Christ?
- What experiences have impacted your life since starting First Place for Health?
- In what ways is Christ working in your life today? In what ways is He meeting your needs?

- How has Christ worked in other members of your First Place for Health group?

Answer the above questions in a few sentences, and then use your answers to help you write your own short personal faith story.

MEMBER SURVEY

We would love to know more about you. Share this form with your leader.

Name _____   Birth date _____

Tell us about your family.

_____

_____

_____

_____

Would you like to receive more information   Yes   No
about our church?

What area of expertise would you be willing to share with our class?

_____

_____

Why did you join First Place for Health?

_____

_____

With notice, would you be willing to lead a Bible study   Yes   No
discussion one week?

Are you comfortable praying out loud?   _____

Would you be willing to assist recording weights and/or   Yes   No
evaluating the Live It Trackers?

Any other comments:

_____

_____

PERSONAL WEIGHT AND MEASUREMENT RECORD

WEEK	WEIGHT	+ OR -	GOAL THIS SESSION	POUNDS TO GOAL
1				
2				
3				
4				
5				
6				
7				
8				
9				
10				
11				
12				

BEGINNING MEASUREMENTS

WAIST_____ HIPS_____ THIGHS_____ CHEST_____

ENDING MEASUREMENTS

WAIST_____ HIPS_____ THIGHS_____ CHEST_____

Very early in the morning, while it was still dark, Jesus got up, left the house and went off to a solitary place, where he prayed.
MARK 1:35

Date: _____

Name: _____

Home Phone: _____

Cell Phone: _____

Email: _____

Personal Prayer Concerns

_____

_____

_____

_____

_____

_____

_____

_____

_____

This form is for prayer requests that are personal to you and your journey in First Place for Health.

Bear with each other and forgive whatever grievances you may have against one another. Forgive as the Lord forgave you.
COLOSSIANS 3:13

Date: _____

Name: _____

Home Phone: _____

Cell Phone: _____

Email: _____

Personal Prayer Concerns

_____

_____

_____

_____

_____

_____

_____

_____

This form is for prayer requests that are personal to you and your journey in First Place for Health. Please complete and have it ready to turn in when you arrive at your group meeting.

I can do all this through him who gives me strength.
PHILIPPIANS 4:13

Date: _____

Name: _____

Home Phone: _____

Cell Phone: _____

Email: _____

Personal Prayer Concerns

_____

_____

_____

_____

_____

_____

_____

_____

This form is for prayer requests that are personal to you and your journey in First Place for Health. Please complete and have it ready to turn in when you arrive at your group meeting.

PRAYER PARTNER   WEEK 4

Be diligent in these matters; give yourself wholly to them, so that
everyone may see your progress.
1 TIMOTHY 4:15

Date: _____

Name: _____

Home Phone: _____

Cell Phone: _____

Email: _____

Personal Prayer Concerns

_____

_____

_____

_____

_____

_____

_____

This form is for prayer requests that are personal to you and your journey in First Place for Health.

The fear of the LORD is the beginning of wisdom; all who follow his precepts
have good understanding. To him belongs eternal praise.
PSALM 111:10

Date: _____

Name: _____

Home Phone: _____

Cell Phone: _____

Email: _____

Personal Prayer Concerns

_____

_____

_____

_____

_____

_____

_____

This form is for prayer requests that are personal to you and your journey in First Place for Health. Please complete and have it ready to turn in when you arrive at your group meeting.

His master replied, "Well done, good and faithful servant! You have been
faithful with a few things; I will put you in charge of many things. Come and
share in your master's happiness!"
MATTHEW 25:23

Date: _____

Name: _____

Home Phone: _____

Cell Phone: _____

Email: _____

Personal Prayer Concerns

_____

_____

_____

_____

_____

_____

_____

_____

This form is for prayer requests that are personal to you and your journey in First Place for Health.
Please complete and have it ready to turn in when you arrive at your group meeting.

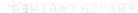

"Love the Lord your God with all your heart and with all your soul and with all your mind and with all your strength." The second is this: "Love your neighbor as yourself." There is no commandment greater than these.
MARK 12:30-31

Date: _____

Name: _____

Home Phone: _____

Cell Phone: _____

Email: _____

Personal Prayer Concerns

_____

_____

_____

_____

_____

_____

_____

This form is for prayer requests that are personal to you and your journey in First Place for Health. Please complete and have it ready to turn in when you arrive at your group meeting.

My kingdom is not of this world.
JOHN 18:36

Date: _____

Name: _____

Home Phone: _____

Cell Phone: _____

Email: _____

Personal Prayer Concern

_____

_____

_____

_____

_____

_____

_____

_____

This form is for prayer requests that are personal to you and your journey in First Place for Health. Please complete and have it ready to turn in when you arrive at your group meeting.

If anyone, then, who knows the good they ought to do and doesn't do it, it is sin for them. JAMES 4:17

Date: _____

Name: _____

Home Phone: _____

Cell Phone: _____

Email: _____

Personal Prayer Concerns

_____

_____

_____

_____

_____

_____

_____

_____

This form is for prayer requests that are personal to you and your journey in First Place for Health. Please complete and have it ready to turn in when you arrive at your group meeting.

PRAYER PARTNER

Be completely humble and gentle; be patient, bearing with one
another in love. Ephesians 4:2

Date: _____

Name:_____

Home Phone: _____

Cell Phone: _____

Email: _____

Personal Prayer Concerns

_____

_____

_____

_____

_____

_____

_____

_____

This form is for prayer requests that are personal to you and your journey in First Place for Health. Please complete and have it ready to turn in when you arrive at your group meeting.

Date: _____

Name: _____

Home Phone: _____

Cell Phone: _____

Email: _____

Personal Prayer Concerns

_____

_____

_____

_____

_____

_____

_____

_____

This form is for prayer requests that are personal to you and your journey in First Place for Health. Please complete and have it ready to turn in when you arrive at your group meeting.

LIVE IT TRACKER

Name: _____

My activity goal for next week:
○ None   ○ <30 min/day   ○ 30-60 min/day

My food goal for next week: _____
_____

Date: _____ Week #: _____

loss/gain _____ Calorie Range: _____

My week at a glance:
○ Great   ○ So-so   ○ Not so great

Activity level:
○ None   ○ <30 min/day   ○ 30-60 min/day

RECOMMENDED DAILY AMOUNT OF FOOD FROM EACH GROUP

GROUP	DAILY CALORIES							
	1300-1400	1500-1600	1700-1800	1900-2000	2100-2200	2300-2400	2500-2600	2700-2800
Fruits	1.5 – 2 c.	1.5 – 2 c.	1.5 – 2 c.	2 – 2.5 c.	2 – 2.5 c.	2.5 – 3.5 c.	3.5 – 4.5 c.	3.5 – 4.5 c.
Vegetables	1.5 – 2 c.	2 – 2.5 c.	2.5 – 3 c.	2.5 – 3 c.	3 – 3.5 c.	3.5 – 4.5 c..	4.5 – 5 c.	4.5 – 5 c.
Grains	5 oz eq.	5-6 oz eq.	6-7 oz eq.	6-7 oz eq.	7-8 oz eq.	8-9 oz eq.	9-10 oz eq.	10-11 oz eq.
Dairy	2-3 c.	3 c.	3 c.	3 c.	3 c.	3 c.	3 c.	3 c.
Protein	4 oz eq.	5 oz eq.	5-5.5 oz eq.	5.5-6.5 oz eq.	6.5-7 oz eq.	7-7.5 oz eq.	7-7.5 oz eq.	7.5-8 oz eq.
Healthy Oils & Other Fats	4 tsp.	5 tsp.	5 tsp.	6 tsp.	6 tsp.	7 tsp.	8 tsp.	8 tsp.
Water & Super Beverages*	Women: 9 c. Men: 13 c.	Women: 9 c. Men: 13 c.	Women: 9 c. Men: 13 c.	Women: 9 c. Men: 13 c.	Women: 9 c. Men: 13 c.	Women: 9 c. Men: 13 c.	Women: 9 c. Men: 13 c.	Women: 9 c. Men: 13 c.

*May count up to 3 cups caffeinated tea or coffee toward goal

DAILY FOOD GROUP TRACKER

GROUP	FRUITS	VEGETABLES	GRAINS	PROTEIN	DAIRY	HEALTHY OILS & OTHER FATS	WATER & SUPER BEVERAGES
1 Estimate Total							
2 Estimate Total							
3 Estimate Total							
4 Estimate Total							
5 Estimate Total							
6 Estimate Total							
7 Estimate Total							

FOOD CHOICES

DAY ❶

Breakfast: _____
Lunch: _____
Dinner: _____
Snacks: _____

PHYSICAL ACTIVITY   steps/miles/minutes: _____

description: _____

SPIRITUAL ACTIVITY

description: _____

FOOD CHOICES DAY ❷

Breakfast: _____
Lunch: _____
Dinner: _____
Snacks: _____

PHYSICAL ACTIVITY   steps/miles/minutes: _____

description: _____

SPIRITUAL ACTIVITY

description: _____

FOOD CHOICES DAY ❸

Breakfast: _____
Lunch: _____
Dinner: _____
Snacks: _____

PHYSICAL ACTIVITY   steps/miles/minutes: _____

description: _____

SPIRITUAL ACTIVITY

description: _____

FOOD CHOICES DAY ❹

Breakfast: _____
Lunch: _____
Dinner: _____
Snacks: _____

PHYSICAL ACTIVITY   steps/miles/minutes: _____

description: _____

SPIRITUAL ACTIVITY

description: _____

FOOD CHOICES DAY ❺

Breakfast: _____
Lunch: _____
Dinner: _____
Snacks: _____

PHYSICAL ACTIVITY   steps/miles/minutes: _____

description: _____

SPIRITUAL ACTIVITY

description: _____

FOOD CHOICES DAY ❻

Breakfast: _____
Lunch: _____
Dinner: _____
Snacks: _____

PHYSICAL ACTIVITY   steps/miles/minutes: _____

description: _____

SPIRITUAL ACTIVITY

description: _____

FOOD CHOICES DAY ❼

Breakfast: _____
Lunch: _____
Dinner: _____
Snacks: _____

PHYSICAL ACTIVITY   steps/miles/minutes: _____

description: _____

SPIRITUAL ACTIVITY

description: _____

LIVE IT TRACKER

Name: _____

Date: _____ Week #: _____

My activity goal for next week:
○ None   ○ <30 min/day   ○ 30-60 min/day

loss/gain _____ Calorie Range: _____

My food goal for next week: _____

My week at a glance:
○ Great   ○ So-so   ○ Not so great

Activity level:
○ None   ○ <30 min/day   ○ 30-60 min/day

RECOMMENDED DAILY AMOUNT OF FOOD FROM EACH GROUP

GROUP	DAILY CALORIES							
......	1300-1400	1500-1600	1700-1800	1900-2000	2100-2200	2300-2400	2500-2600	2700-2800
Fruits	1.5 – 2 c.	1.5 – 2 c.	1.5 – 2 c.	2 – 2.5 c.	2 – 2.5 c.	2.5 – 3.5 c.	3.5 – 4.5 c.	3.5 – 4.5 c.
Vegetables	1.5 – 2 c.	2 – 2.5 c.	2.5 – 3 c.	2.5 – 3 c.	3 – 3.5 c.	3.5 – 4.5 c..	4.5 – 5 c.	4.5 – 5 c.
Grains	5 oz eq.	5-6 oz eq.	6-7 oz eq.	6-7 oz eq.	7-8 oz eq.	8-9 oz eq.	9-10 oz eq.	10-11 oz eq.
Dairy	2-3 c.	3 c.	3 c.	3 c.	3 c.	3 c.	3 c.	3 c.
Protein	4 oz eq.	5 oz eq.	5-5.5 oz eq.	5.5-6.5 oz eq.	6.5-7 oz eq.	7-7.5 oz eq.	7-7.5 oz eq.	7.5-8 oz eq.
Healthy Oils & Other Fats	4 tsp.	5 tsp.	5 tsp.	6 tsp.	6 tsp.	7 tsp.	8 tsp.	8 tsp.
Water & Super Beverages*	Women: 9 c. Men: 13 c.	Women: 9 c. Men: 13 c.	Women: 9 c. Men: 13 c.	Women: 9 c. Men: 13 c.	Women: 9 c. Men: 13 c.	Women: 9 c. Men: 13 c.	Women: 9 c. Men: 13 c.	Women: 9 c. Men: 13 c.

*May count up to 3 cups caffeinated tea or coffee toward goal

DAILY FOOD GROUP TRACKER

GROUP	FRUITS	VEGETABLES	GRAINS	PROTEIN	DAIRY	HEALTHY OILS & OTHER FATS	WATER & SUPER BEVERAGES
1 Estimate Total							
2 Estimate Total							
3 Estimate Total							
4 Estimate Total							
5 Estimate Total							
6 Estimate Total							
7 Estimate Total							

FOOD CHOICES

DAY 1

Breakfast: _____
Lunch: _____
Dinner: _____
Snacks: _____

PHYSICAL ACTIVITY   steps/miles/minutes: _____
description: _____

SPIRITUAL ACTIVITY
description: _____

FOOD CHOICES

DAY 2

Breakfast: _____

Lunch: _____

Dinner: _____

Snacks: _____

PHYSICAL ACTIVITY steps/miles/minutes: _____

description: _____

SPIRITUAL ACTIVITY

description: _____

FOOD CHOICES

DAY 3

Breakfast: _____

Lunch: _____

Dinner: _____

Snacks: _____

PHYSICAL ACTIVITY steps/miles/minutes: _____

description: _____

SPIRITUAL ACTIVITY

description: _____

FOOD CHOICES

DAY 4

Breakfast: _____

Lunch: _____

Dinner: _____

Snacks: _____

PHYSICAL ACTIVITY steps/miles/minutes: _____

description: _____

SPIRITUAL ACTIVITY

description: _____

FOOD CHOICES

DAY 5

Breakfast: _____

Lunch: _____

Dinner: _____

Snacks: _____

PHYSICAL ACTIVITY steps/miles/minutes: _____

description: _____

SPIRITUAL ACTIVITY

description: _____

FOOD CHOICES

DAY 6

Breakfast: _____

Lunch: _____

Dinner: _____

Snacks: _____

PHYSICAL ACTIVITY steps/miles/minutes: _____

description: _____

SPIRITUAL ACTIVITY

description: _____

FOOD CHOICES

DAY 7

Breakfast: _____

Lunch: _____

Dinner: _____

Snacks: _____

PHYSICAL ACTIVITY steps/miles/minutes: _____

description: _____

SPIRITUAL ACTIVITY

description: _____

LIVE IT TRACKER

Name: _____

My activity goal for next week:
○ None ○ <30 min/day ○ 30-60 min/day

My food goal for next week: _____
_____

Date: _____ Week #: _____

loss/gain _____ Calorie Range: _____

My week at a glance:
○ Great ○ So-so ○ Not so great

Activity level:
○ None ○ <30 min/day ○ 30-60 min/day

RECOMMENDED DAILY AMOUNT OF FOOD FROM EACH GROUP

GROUP	DAILY CALORIES							
	1300-1400	1500-1600	1700-1800	1900-2000	2100-2200	2300-2400	2500-2600	2700-2800
Fruits	1.5 – 2 c.	1.5 – 2 c.	1.5 – 2 c.	2 – 2.5 c.	2 – 2.5 c.	2.5 – 3.5 c.	3.5 – 4.5 c.	3.5 – 4.5 c.
Vegetables	1.5 – 2 c.	2 – 2.5 c.	2.5 – 3 c.	2.5 – 3 c.	3 – 3.5 c.	3.5 – 4.5 c..	4.5 – 5 c.	4.5 – 5 c.
Grains	5 oz eq.	5-6 oz eq.	6-7 oz eq.	6-7 oz eq.	7-8 oz eq.	8-9 oz eq.	9-10 oz eq.	10-11 oz eq.
Dairy	2-3 c.	3 c.	3 c.	3 c.	3 c.	3 c.	3 c.	3 c.
Protein	4 oz eq.	5 oz eq.	5-5.5 oz eq.	5.5-6.5 oz eq.	6.5-7 oz eq.	7-7.5 oz eq.	7-7.5 oz eq.	7.5-8 oz eq.
Healthy Oils & Other Fats	4 tsp.	5 tsp.	5 tsp.	6 tsp.	6 tsp.	7 tsp.	8 tsp.	8 tsp.
Water & Super Beverages*	Women: 9 c. Men: 13 c.	Women: 9 c. Men: 13 c.	Women: 9 c. Men: 13 c.	Women: 9 c. Men: 13 c.	Women: 9 c. Men: 13 c.	Women: 9 c. Men: 13 c.	Women: 9 c. Men: 13 c.	Women: 9 c. Men: 13 c.

*May count up to 3 cups caffeinated tea or coffee toward goal

DAILY FOOD GROUP TRACKER

GROUP	FRUITS	VEGETABLES	GRAINS	PROTEIN	DAIRY	HEALTHY OILS & OTHER FATS	WATER & SUPER BEVERAGES
① Estimate Total							
② Estimate Total							
③ Estimate Total							
④ Estimate Total							
⑤ Estimate Total							
⑥ Estimate Total							
⑦ Estimate Total							

FOOD CHOICES

DAY ❶

Breakfast: _____
Lunch: _____
Dinner: _____
Snacks: _____

PHYSICAL ACTIVITY   steps/miles/minutes: _____

description: _____
_____

SPIRITUAL ACTIVITY

description: _____
_____

FOOD CHOICES   DAY ➋

Breakfast: _____
Lunch: _____
Dinner: _____
Snacks: _____

PHYSICAL ACTIVITY   steps/miles/minutes: _____   ### SPIRITUAL ACTIVITY
description: _____   description: _____

FOOD CHOICES   DAY ➌

Breakfast: _____
Lunch: _____
Dinner: _____
Snacks: _____

PHYSICAL ACTIVITY   steps/miles/minutes: _____   ### SPIRITUAL ACTIVITY
description: _____   description: _____

FOOD CHOICES   DAY ➍

Breakfast: _____
Lunch: _____
Dinner: _____
Snacks: _____

PHYSICAL ACTIVITY   steps/miles/minutes: _____   ### SPIRITUAL ACTIVITY
description: _____   description: _____

FOOD CHOICES   DAY ➎

Breakfast: _____
Lunch: _____
Dinner: _____
Snacks: _____

PHYSICAL ACTIVITY   steps/miles/minutes: _____   ### SPIRITUAL ACTIVITY
description: _____   description: _____

FOOD CHOICES   DAY ➏

Breakfast: _____
Lunch: _____
Dinner: _____
Snacks: _____

PHYSICAL ACTIVITY   steps/miles/minutes: _____   ### SPIRITUAL ACTIVITY
description: _____   description: _____

FOOD CHOICES   DAY ➐

Breakfast: _____
Lunch: _____
Dinner: _____
Snacks: _____

PHYSICAL ACTIVITY   steps/miles/minutes: _____   ### SPIRITUAL ACTIVITY
description: _____   description: _____

LIVE IT TRACKER

Name: _____

My activity goal for next week:
○ None   ○ <30 min/day   ○ 30-60 min/day

My food goal for next week: _____
_____

Date: _____ Week #: _____

loss/gain _____ Calorie Range: _____

My week at a glance:
○ Great   ○ So-so   ○ Not so great

Activity level:
○ None   ○ <30 min/day   ○ 30-60 min/day

RECOMMENDED DAILY AMOUNT OF FOOD FROM EACH GROUP

GROUP	DAILY CALORIES							
	1300-1400	1500-1600	1700-1800	1900-2000	2100-2200	2300-2400	2500-2600	2700-2800
Fruits	1.5 – 2 c.	1.5 – 2 c.	1.5 – 2 c.	2 – 2.5 c.	2 – 2.5 c.	2.5 – 3.5 c.	3.5 – 4.5 c.	3.5 – 4.5 c.
Vegetables	1.5 – 2 c.	2 – 2.5 c.	2.5 – 3 c.	2.5 – 3 c.	3 – 3.5 c.	3.5 – 4.5 c..	4.5 – 5 c.	4.5 – 5 c.
Grains	5 oz eq.	5-6 oz eq.	6-7 oz eq.	6-7 oz eq.	7-8 oz eq.	8-9 oz eq.	9-10 oz eq.	10-11 oz eq.
Dairy	2-3 c.	3 c.	3 c.	3 c.	3 c.	3 c.	3 c.	3 c.
Protein	4 oz eq.	5 oz eq.	5-5.5 oz eq.	5.5-6.5 oz eq.	6.5-7 oz eq.	7-7.5 oz eq.	7-7.5 oz eq.	7.5-8 oz eq.
Healthy Oils & Other Fats	4 tsp.	5 tsp.	5 tsp.	6 tsp.	6 tsp.	7 tsp.	8 tsp.	8 tsp.
Water & Super Beverages*	Women: 9 c. Men: 13 c.	Women: 9 c. Men: 13 c.	Women: 9 c. Men: 13 c.	Women: 9 c. Men: 13 c.	Women: 9 c. Men: 13 c.	Women: 9 c. Men: 13 c.	Women: 9 c. Men: 13 c.	Women: 9 c. Men: 13 c.

*May count up to 3 cups caffeinated tea or coffee toward goal

DAILY FOOD GROUP TRACKER

GROUP	FRUITS	VEGETABLES	GRAINS	PROTEIN	DAIRY	HEALTHY OILS & OTHER FATS	WATER & SUPER BEVERAGES
1 Estimate Total							
2 Estimate Total							
3 Estimate Total							
4 Estimate Total							
5 Estimate Total							
6 Estimate Total							
7 Estimate Total							

FOOD CHOICES

DAY ❶

Breakfast: _____
Lunch: _____
Dinner: _____
Snacks: _____

PHYSICAL ACTIVITY   steps/miles/minutes: _____

description: _____
_____

SPIRITUAL ACTIVITY

description: _____
_____

FOOD CHOICES DAY ❷

Breakfast: _____
Lunch: _____
Dinner: _____
Snacks: _____

PHYSICAL ACTIVITY   steps/miles/minutes: _____   ### SPIRITUAL ACTIVITY

description: _____   description: _____

FOOD CHOICES DAY ❸

Breakfast: _____
Lunch: _____
Dinner: _____
Snacks: _____

PHYSICAL ACTIVITY   steps/miles/minutes: _____   ### SPIRITUAL ACTIVITY

description: _____   description: _____

FOOD CHOICES DAY ❹

Breakfast: _____
Lunch: _____
Dinner: _____
Snacks: _____

PHYSICAL ACTIVITY   steps/miles/minutes: _____   ### SPIRITUAL ACTIVITY

description: _____   description: _____

FOOD CHOICES DAY ❺

Breakfast: _____
Lunch: _____
Dinner: _____
Snacks: _____

PHYSICAL ACTIVITY   steps/miles/minutes: _____   ### SPIRITUAL ACTIVITY

description: _____   description: _____

FOOD CHOICES DAY ❻

Breakfast: _____
Lunch: _____
Dinner: _____
Snacks: _____

PHYSICAL ACTIVITY   steps/miles/minutes: _____   ### SPIRITUAL ACTIVITY

description: _____   description: _____

FOOD CHOICES DAY ❼

Breakfast: _____
Lunch: _____
Dinner: _____
Snacks: _____

PHYSICAL ACTIVITY   steps/miles/minutes: _____   ### SPIRITUAL ACTIVITY

description: _____   description: _____

LIVE IT TRACKER

Name: _____

My activity goal for next week:
○ None   ○ <30 min/day   ○ 30-60 min/day

My food goal for next week: _____
_____

Date: _____ Week #: _____

loss/gain _____ Calorie Range: _____

My week at a glance:
○ Great   ○ So-so   ○ Not so great

Activity level:
○ None   ○ <30 min/day   ○ 30-60 min/day

RECOMMENDED DAILY AMOUNT OF FOOD FROM EACH GROUP

GROUP	DAILY CALORIES							
......	1300-1400	1500-1600	1700-1800	1900-2000	2100-2200	2300-2400	2500-2600	2700-2800
Fruits	1.5 – 2 c.	1.5 – 2 c.	1.5 – 2 c.	2 – 2.5 c.	2 – 2.5 c.	2.5 – 3.5 c.	3.5 – 4.5 c.	3.5 – 4.5 c.
Vegetables	1.5 – 2 c.	2 – 2.5 c.	2.5 – 3 c.	2.5 – 3 c.	3 – 3.5 c.	3.5 – 4.5 c..	4.5 – 5 c.	4.5 – 5 c.
Grains	5 oz eq.	5-6 oz eq.	6-7 oz eq.	6-7 oz eq.	7-8 oz eq.	8-9 oz eq.	9-10 oz eq.	10-11 oz eq.
Dairy	2-3 c.	3 c.	3 c.	3 c.	3 c.	3 c.	3 c.	3 c.
Protein	4 oz eq.	5 oz eq.	5-5.5 oz eq.	5.5-6.5 oz eq.	6.5-7 oz eq.	7-7.5 oz eq.	7-7.5 oz eq.	7.5-8 oz eq.
Healthy Oils & Other Fats	4 tsp.	5 tsp.	5 tsp.	6 tsp.	6 tsp.	7 tsp.	8 tsp.	8 tsp.
Water & Super Beverages*	Women: 9 c. Men: 13 c.	Women: 9 c. Men: 13 c.	Women: 9 c. Men: 13 c.	Women: 9 c. Men: 13 c.	Women: 9 c. Men: 13 c.	Women: 9 c. Men: 13 c.	Women: 9 c. Men: 13 c.	Women: 9 c. Men: 13 c.

*May count up to 3 cups caffeinated tea or coffee toward goal

DAILY FOOD GROUP TRACKER

GROUP	FRUITS	VEGETABLES	GRAINS	PROTEIN	DAIRY	HEALTHY OILS & OTHER FATS	WATER & SUPER BEVERAGES
1 Estimate Total							
2 Estimate Total							
3 Estimate Total							
4 Estimate Total							
5 Estimate Total							
6 Estimate Total							
7 Estimate Total							

FOOD CHOICES

DAY ❶

Breakfast: _____
Lunch: _____
Dinner: _____
Snacks: _____

PHYSICAL ACTIVITY   steps/miles/minutes: _____
description: _____
_____

SPIRITUAL ACTIVITY
description: _____
_____

FOOD CHOICES

DAY 2

Breakfast: _____
Lunch: _____
Dinner: _____
Snacks: _____

PHYSICAL ACTIVITY   steps/miles/minutes: _____

description: _____

SPIRITUAL ACTIVITY

description: _____

FOOD CHOICES

DAY 3

Breakfast: _____
Lunch: _____
Dinner: _____
Snacks: _____

PHYSICAL ACTIVITY   steps/miles/minutes: _____

description: _____

SPIRITUAL ACTIVITY

description: _____

FOOD CHOICES

DAY 4

Breakfast: _____
Lunch: _____
Dinner: _____
Snacks: _____

PHYSICAL ACTIVITY   steps/miles/minutes: _____

description: _____

SPIRITUAL ACTIVITY

description: _____

FOOD CHOICES

DAY 5

Breakfast: _____
Lunch: _____
Dinner: _____
Snacks: _____

PHYSICAL ACTIVITY   steps/miles/minutes: _____

description: _____

SPIRITUAL ACTIVITY

description: _____

FOOD CHOICES

DAY 6

Breakfast: _____
Lunch: _____
Dinner: _____
Snacks: _____

PHYSICAL ACTIVITY   steps/miles/minutes: _____

description: _____

SPIRITUAL ACTIVITY

description: _____

FOOD CHOICES

DAY 7

Breakfast: _____
Lunch: _____
Dinner: _____
Snacks: _____

PHYSICAL ACTIVITY   steps/miles/minutes: _____

description: _____

SPIRITUAL ACTIVITY

description: _____

LIVE IT TRACKER

Name: _____

Date: _____ Week #: _____

My activity goal for next week:
○ None   ○ <30 min/day   ○ 30-60 min/day

My food goal for next week: _____
_____

loss / gain _____ Calorie Range: _____

My week at a glance:
○ Great   ○ So-so   ○ Not so great

Activity level:
○ None   ○ <30 min/day   ○ 30-60 min/day

RECOMMENDED DAILY AMOUNT OF FOOD FROM EACH GROUP

GROUP	DAILY CALORIES							
	1300-1400	1500-1600	1700-1800	1900-2000	2100-2200	2300-2400	2500-2600	2700-2800
Fruits	1.5 – 2 c.	1.5 – 2 c.	1.5 – 2 c.	2 – 2.5 c.	2 – 2.5 c.	2.5 – 3.5 c.	3.5 – 4.5 c.	3.5 – 4.5 c.
Vegetables	1.5 – 2 c.	2 – 2.5 c.	2.5 – 3 c.	2.5 – 3 c.	3 – 3.5 c.	3.5 – 4.5 c..	4.5 – 5 c.	4.5 – 5 c.
Grains	5 oz eq.	5-6 oz eq.	6-7 oz eq.	6-7 oz eq.	7-8 oz eq.	8-9 oz eq.	9-10 oz eq.	10-11 oz eq.
Dairy	2-3 c.	3 c.	3 c.	3 c.	3 c.	3 c.	3 c.	3 c.
Protein	4 oz eq.	5 oz eq.	5-5.5 oz eq.	5.5-6.5 oz eq.	6.5-7 oz eq.	7-7.5 oz eq.	7-7.5 oz eq.	7.5-8 oz eq.
Healthy Oils & Other Fats	4 tsp.	5 tsp.	5 tsp.	6 tsp.	6 tsp.	7 tsp.	8 tsp.	8 tsp.
Water & Super Beverages*	Women: 9 c. Men: 13 c.	Women: 9 c. Men: 13 c.	Women: 9 c. Men: 13 c.	Women: 9 c. Men: 13 c.	Women: 9 c. Men: 13 c.	Women: 9 c. Men: 13 c.	Women: 9 c. Men: 13 c.	Women: 9 c. Men: 13 c.

*May count up to 3 cups caffeinated tea or coffee toward goal

DAILY FOOD GROUP TRACKER

	GROUP	FRUITS	VEGETABLES	GRAINS	PROTEIN	DAIRY	HEALTHY OILS & OTHER FATS	WATER & SUPER BEVERAGES
1	Estimate Total							
2	Estimate Total							
3	Estimate Total							
4	Estimate Total							
5	Estimate Total							
6	Estimate Total							
7	Estimate Total							

FOOD CHOICES   DAY ❶

Breakfast: _____
Lunch: _____
Dinner: _____
Snacks: _____

PHYSICAL ACTIVITY   steps/miles/minutes: _____

description: _____

SPIRITUAL ACTIVITY

description: _____

215

FOOD CHOICES

DAY 2

Breakfast: _____

Lunch: _____

Dinner: _____

Snacks: _____

PHYSICAL ACTIVITY   steps/miles/minutes: _____

description: _____

SPIRITUAL ACTIVITY

description: _____

FOOD CHOICES

DAY 3

Breakfast: _____

Lunch: _____

Dinner: _____

Snacks: _____

PHYSICAL ACTIVITY   steps/miles/minutes: _____

description: _____

SPIRITUAL ACTIVITY

description: _____

FOOD CHOICES

DAY 4

Breakfast: _____

Lunch: _____

Dinner: _____

Snacks: _____

PHYSICAL ACTIVITY   steps/miles/minutes: _____

description: _____

SPIRITUAL ACTIVITY

description: _____

FOOD CHOICES

DAY 5

Breakfast: _____

Lunch: _____

Dinner: _____

Snacks: _____

PHYSICAL ACTIVITY   steps/miles/minutes: _____

description: _____

SPIRITUAL ACTIVITY

description: _____

FOOD CHOICES

DAY 6

Breakfast: _____

Lunch: _____

Dinner: _____

Snacks: _____

PHYSICAL ACTIVITY   steps/miles/minutes: _____

description: _____

SPIRITUAL ACTIVITY

description: _____

FOOD CHOICES

DAY 7

Breakfast: _____

Lunch: _____

Dinner: _____

Snacks: _____

PHYSICAL ACTIVITY   steps/miles/minutes: _____

description: _____

SPIRITUAL ACTIVITY

description: _____

LIVE IT TRACKER

Name: _____

Date: _____ Week #: _____

My activity goal for next week:
- ○ None ○ <30 min/day ○ 30-60 min/day

loss /gain _____ Calorie Range: _____

My food goal for next week: _____
_____

My week at a glance:
- ○ Great ○ So-so ○ Not so great

Activity level:
- ○ None ○ <30 min/day ○ 30-60 min/day

RECOMMENDED DAILY AMOUNT OF FOOD FROM EACH GROUP

DAILY CALORIES

GROUP	1300-1400	1500-1600	1700-1800	1900-2000	2100-2200	2300-2400	2500-2600	2700-2800
Fruits	1.5 – 2 c.	1.5 – 2 c.	1.5 – 2 c.	2 – 2.5 c.	2 – 2.5 c.	2.5 – 3.5 c.	3.5 – 4.5 c.	3.5 – 4.5 c.
Vegetables	1.5 – 2 c.	2 – 2.5 c.	2.5 – 3 c.	2.5 – 3 c.	3 – 3.5 c.	3.5 – 4.5 c..	4.5 – 5 c.	4.5 – 5 c.
Grains	5 oz eq.	5-6 oz eq.	6-7 oz eq.	6-7 oz eq.	7-8 oz eq.	8-9 oz eq.	9-10 oz eq.	10-11 oz eq.
Dairy	2-3 c.	3 c.	3 c.	3 c.	3 c.	3 c.	3 c.	3 c.
Protein	4 oz eq.	5 oz eq.	5-5.5 oz eq.	5.5-6.5 oz eq.	6.5-7 oz eq.	7-7.5 oz eq.	7-7.5 oz eq.	7.5-8 oz eq.
Healthy Oils & Other Fats	4 tsp.	5 tsp.	5 tsp.	6 tsp.	6 tsp.	7 tsp.	8 tsp.	8 tsp.
Water & Super Beverages*	Women: 9 c. Men: 13 c.	Women: 9 c. Men: 13 c.	Women: 9 c. Men: 13 c.	Women: 9 c. Men: 13 c.	Women: 9 c. Men: 13 c.	Women: 9 c. Men: 13 c.	Women: 9 c. Men: 13 c.	Women: 9 c. Men: 13 c.

*May count up to 3 cups caffeinated tea or coffee toward goal

DAILY FOOD GROUP TRACKER

GROUP	FRUITS	VEGETABLES	GRAINS	PROTEIN	DAIRY	HEALTHY OILS & OTHER FATS	WATER & SUPER BEVERAGES
1 Estimate Total							
2 Estimate Total							
3 Estimate Total							
4 Estimate Total							
5 Estimate Total							
6 Estimate Total							
7 Estimate Total							

FOOD CHOICES

DAY 1

Breakfast: _____
Lunch: _____
Dinner: _____
Snacks: _____

PHYSICAL ACTIVITY   steps/miles/minutes: _____

description: _____
_____

SPIRITUAL ACTIVITY

description: _____
_____

FOOD CHOICES

DAY ❷

Breakfast: _____

Lunch: _____

Dinner: _____

Snacks: _____

PHYSICAL ACTIVITY   steps/miles/minutes: _____

description: _____

SPIRITUAL ACTIVITY

description: _____

FOOD CHOICES

DAY ❸

Breakfast: _____

Lunch: _____

Dinner: _____

Snacks: _____

PHYSICAL ACTIVITY   steps/miles/minutes: _____

description: _____

SPIRITUAL ACTIVITY

description: _____

FOOD CHOICES

DAY ❹

Breakfast: _____

Lunch: _____

Dinner: _____

Snacks: _____

PHYSICAL ACTIVITY   steps/miles/minutes: _____

description: _____

SPIRITUAL ACTIVITY

description: _____

FOOD CHOICES

DAY ❺

Breakfast: _____

Lunch: _____

Dinner: _____

Snacks: _____

PHYSICAL ACTIVITY   steps/miles/minutes: _____

description: _____

SPIRITUAL ACTIVITY

description: _____

FOOD CHOICES

DAY ❻

Breakfast: _____

Lunch: _____

Dinner: _____

Snacks: _____

PHYSICAL ACTIVITY   steps/miles/minutes: _____

description: _____

SPIRITUAL ACTIVITY

description: _____

FOOD CHOICES

DAY ❼

Breakfast: _____

Lunch: _____

Dinner: _____

Snacks: _____

PHYSICAL ACTIVITY   steps/miles/minutes: _____

description: _____

SPIRITUAL ACTIVITY

description: _____

LIVE IT TRACKER

Name: _____

Date: _____ Week #: _____

My activity goal for next week:
○ None   ○ <30 min/day   ○ 30-60 min/day

loss /gain _____ Calorie Range: _____

My week at a glance:
○ Great   ○ So-so   ○ Not so great

My food goal for next week: _____
_____

Activity level:
○ None   ○ <30 min/day   ○ 30-60 min/day

RECOMMENDED DAILY AMOUNT OF FOOD FROM EACH GROUP

GROUP	DAILY CALORIES							
......	1300-1400	1500-1600	1700-1800	1900-2000	2100-2200	2300-2400	2500-2600	2700-2800
Fruits	1.5 – 2 c.	1.5 – 2 c.	1.5 – 2 c.	2 – 2.5 c.	2 – 2.5 c.	2.5 – 3.5 c.	3.5 – 4.5 c.	3.5 – 4.5 c.
Vegetables	1.5 – 2 c.	2 – 2.5 c.	2.5 – 3 c.	2.5 – 3 c.	3 – 3.5 c.	3.5 – 4.5 c..	4.5 – 5 c.	4.5 – 5 c.
Grains	5 oz eq.	5-6 oz eq.	6-7 oz eq.	6-7 oz eq.	7-8 oz eq.	8-9 oz eq.	9-10 oz eq.	10-11 oz eq.
Dairy	2-3 c.	3 c.	3 c.	3 c.	3 c.	3 c.	3 c.	3 c.
Protein	4 oz eq.	5 oz eq.	5-5.5 oz eq.	5.5-6.5 oz eq.	6.5-7 oz eq.	7-7.5 oz eq.	7-7.5 oz eq.	7.5-8 oz eq.
Healthy Oils & Other Fats	4 tsp.	5 tsp.	5 tsp.	6 tsp.	6 tsp.	7 tsp.	8 tsp.	8 tsp.
Water & Super Beverages*	Women: 9 c. Men: 13 c.	Women: 9 c. Men: 13 c.	Women: 9 c. Men: 13 c.	Women: 9 c. Men: 13 c.	Women: 9 c. Men: 13 c.	Women: 9 c. Men: 13 c.	Women: 9 c. Men: 13 c.	Women: 9 c. Men: 13 c.

*May count up to 3 cups caffeinated tea or coffee toward goal

DAILY FOOD GROUP TRACKER

GROUP	FRUITS	VEGETABLES	GRAINS	PROTEIN	DAIRY	HEALTHY OILS & OTHER FATS	WATER & SUPER BEVERAGES
1 Estimate Total							
2 Estimate Total							
3 Estimate Total							
4 Estimate Total							
5 Estimate Total							
6 Estimate Total							
7 Estimate Total							

FOOD CHOICES

DAY 1

Breakfast: _____
Lunch: _____
Dinner: _____
Snacks: _____

PHYSICAL ACTIVITY   steps/miles/minutes: _____

description: _____

SPIRITUAL ACTIVITY

description: _____

FOOD CHOICES DAY ❷

Breakfast: _____
Lunch: _____
Dinner: _____
Snacks: _____

PHYSICAL ACTIVITY   steps/miles/minutes:_____   **SPIRITUAL ACTIVITY**

description: _____   description: _____

FOOD CHOICES DAY ❸

Breakfast: _____
Lunch: _____
Dinner: _____
Snacks: _____

PHYSICAL ACTIVITY   steps/miles/minutes:_____   **SPIRITUAL ACTIVITY**

description: _____   description: _____

FOOD CHOICES DAY ❹

Breakfast: _____
Lunch: _____
Dinner: _____
Snacks: _____

PHYSICAL ACTIVITY   steps/miles/minutes:_____   **SPIRITUAL ACTIVITY**

description: _____   description: _____

FOOD CHOICES DAY ❺

Breakfast: _____
Lunch: _____
Dinner: _____
Snacks: _____

PHYSICAL ACTIVITY   steps/miles/minutes:_____   **SPIRITUAL ACTIVITY**

description: _____   description: _____

FOOD CHOICES DAY ❻

Breakfast: _____
Lunch: _____
Dinner: _____
Snacks: _____

PHYSICAL ACTIVITY   steps/miles/minutes:_____   **SPIRITUAL ACTIVITY**

description: _____   description: _____

FOOD CHOICES DAY ❼

Breakfast: _____
Lunch: _____
Dinner: _____
Snacks: _____

PHYSICAL ACTIVITY   steps/miles/minutes:_____   **SPIRITUAL ACTIVITY**

description: _____   description: _____

LIVE IT TRACKER

Name: _____

My activity goal for next week:
○ None   ○ <30 min/day   ○ 30-60 min/day

My food goal for next week: _____
_____

Date: _____ Week #: _____

loss / gain _____ Calorie Range: _____

My week at a glance:
○ Great   ○ So-so   ○ Not so great

Activity level:
○ None   ○ <30 min/day   ○ 30-60 min/day

RECOMMENDED DAILY AMOUNT OF FOOD FROM EACH GROUP

GROUP	DAILY CALORIES							
	1300-1400	1500-1600	1700-1800	1900-2000	2100-2200	2300-2400	2500-2600	2700-2800
Fruits	1.5 – 2 c.	1.5 – 2 c.	1.5 – 2 c.	2 – 2.5 c.	2 – 2.5 c.	2.5 – 3.5 c.	3.5 – 4.5 c.	3.5 – 4.5 c.
Vegetables	1.5 – 2 c.	2 – 2.5 c.	2.5 – 3 c.	2.5 – 3 c.	3 – 3.5 c.	3.5 – 4.5 c..	4.5 – 5 c.	4.5 – 5 c.
Grains	5 oz eq.	5-6 oz eq.	6-7 oz eq.	6-7 oz eq.	7-8 oz eq.	8-9 oz eq.	9-10 oz eq.	10-11 oz eq.
Dairy	2-3 c.	3 c.	3 c.	3 c.	3 c.	3 c.	3 c.	3 c.
Protein	4 oz eq.	5 oz eq.	5-5.5 oz eq.	5.5-6.5 oz eq.	6.5-7 oz eq.	7-7.5 oz eq.	7-7.5 oz eq.	7.5-8 oz eq.
Healthy Oils & Other Fats	4 tsp.	5 tsp.	5 tsp.	6 tsp.	6 tsp.	7 tsp.	8 tsp.	8 tsp.
Water & Super Beverages*	Women: 9 c. Men: 13 c.	Women: 9 c. Men: 13 c.	Women: 9 c. Men: 13 c.	Women: 9 c. Men: 13 c.	Women: 9 c. Men: 13 c.	Women: 9 c. Men: 13 c.	Women: 9 c. Men: 13 c.	Women: 9 c. Men: 13 c.

*May count up to 3 cups caffeinated tea or coffee toward goal

DAILY FOOD GROUP TRACKER

GROUP	FRUITS	VEGETABLES	GRAINS	PROTEIN	DAIRY	HEALTHY OILS & OTHER FATS	WATER & SUPER BEVERAGES
1 Estimate Total							
2 Estimate Total							
3 Estimate Total							
4 Estimate Total							
5 Estimate Total							
6 Estimate Total							
7 Estimate Total							

FOOD CHOICES

DAY ❶

Breakfast: _____
Lunch: _____
Dinner: _____
Snacks: _____

PHYSICAL ACTIVITY   steps/miles/minutes: _____

description: _____

SPIRITUAL ACTIVITY

description: _____

FOOD CHOICES   DAY ❷

Breakfast: _____
Lunch: _____
Dinner: _____
Snacks: _____

PHYSICAL ACTIVITY   steps/miles/minutes: _____   **SPIRITUAL ACTIVITY**

description: _____   description: _____

FOOD CHOICES   DAY ❸

Breakfast: _____
Lunch: _____
Dinner: _____
Snacks: _____

PHYSICAL ACTIVITY   steps/miles/minutes: _____   **SPIRITUAL ACTIVITY**

description: _____   description: _____

FOOD CHOICES   DAY ❹

Breakfast: _____
Lunch: _____
Dinner: _____
Snacks: _____

PHYSICAL ACTIVITY   steps/miles/minutes: _____   **SPIRITUAL ACTIVITY**

description: _____   description: _____

FOOD CHOICES   DAY ❺

Breakfast: _____
Lunch: _____
Dinner: _____
Snacks: _____

PHYSICAL ACTIVITY   steps/miles/minutes: _____   **SPIRITUAL ACTIVITY**

description: _____   description: _____

FOOD CHOICES   DAY ❻

Breakfast: _____
Lunch: _____
Dinner: _____
Snacks: _____

PHYSICAL ACTIVITY   steps/miles/minutes: _____   **SPIRITUAL ACTIVITY**

description: _____   description: _____

FOOD CHOICES   DAY ❼

Breakfast: _____
Lunch: _____
Dinner: _____
Snacks: _____

PHYSICAL ACTIVITY   steps/miles/minutes: _____   **SPIRITUAL ACTIVITY**

description: _____   description: _____

LIVE IT TRACKER

Name: _____

Date: _____ Week #: _____

My activity goal for next week:
○ None   ○ <30 min/day   ○ 30-60 min/day

My food goal for next week: _____
_____

loss /gain _____   Calorie Range: _____

My week at a glance:
○ Great   ○ So-so   ○ Not so great

Activity level:
○ None   ○ <30 min/day   ○ 30-60 min/day

RECOMMENDED DAILY AMOUNT OF FOOD FROM EACH GROUP

GROUP	DAILY CALORIES							
	1300-1400	1500-1600	1700-1800	1900-2000	2100-2200	2300-2400	2500-2600	2700-2800
Fruits	1.5 – 2 c.	1.5 – 2 c.	1.5 – 2 c.	2 – 2.5 c.	2 – 2.5 c.	2.5 – 3.5 c.	3.5 – 4.5 c.	3.5 – 4.5 c.
Vegetables	1.5 – 2 c.	2 – 2.5 c.	2.5 – 3 c.	2.5 – 3 c.	3 – 3.5 c.	3.5 – 4.5 c..	4.5 – 5 c.	4.5 – 5 c.
Grains	5 oz eq.	5-6 oz eq.	6-7 oz eq.	6-7 oz eq.	7-8 oz eq.	8-9 oz eq.	9-10 oz eq.	10-11 oz eq.
Dairy	2-3 c.	3 c.	3 c.	3 c.	3 c.	3 c.	3 c.	3 c.
Protein	4 oz eq.	5 oz eq.	5-5.5 oz eq.	5.5-6.5 oz eq.	6.5-7 oz eq.	7-7.5 oz eq.	7-7.5 oz eq.	7.5-8 oz eq.
Healthy Oils & Other Fats	4 tsp.	5 tsp.	5 tsp.	6 tsp.	6 tsp.	7 tsp.	8 tsp.	8 tsp.
Water & Super Beverages*	Women: 9 c. Men: 13 c.	Women: 9 c. Men: 13 c.	Women: 9 c. Men: 13 c.	Women: 9 c. Men: 13 c.	Women: 9 c. Men: 13 c.	Women: 9 c. Men: 13 c.	Women: 9 c. Men: 13 c.	Women: 9 c. Men: 13 c.

*May count up to 3 cups caffeinated tea or coffee toward goal

DAILY FOOD GROUP TRACKER

GROUP	FRUITS	VEGETABLES	GRAINS	PROTEIN	DAIRY	HEALTHY OILS & OTHER FATS	WATER & SUPER BEVERAGES
1 Estimate Total							
2 Estimate Total							
3 Estimate Total							
4 Estimate Total							
5 Estimate Total							
6 Estimate Total							
7 Estimate Total							

FOOD CHOICES

DAY 1

Breakfast: _____
Lunch: _____
Dinner: _____
Snacks: _____

PHYSICAL ACTIVITY   steps/miles/minutes: _____
description: _____

SPIRITUAL ACTIVITY
description: _____

FOOD CHOICES

DAY 2

Breakfast: _____

Lunch: _____

Dinner: _____

Snacks: _____

PHYSICAL ACTIVITY   steps/miles/minutes: _____ | **SPIRITUAL ACTIVITY**

description: _____ | description: _____

FOOD CHOICES

DAY 3

Breakfast: _____

Lunch: _____

Dinner: _____

Snacks: _____

PHYSICAL ACTIVITY   steps/miles/minutes: _____ | **SPIRITUAL ACTIVITY**

description: _____ | description: _____

FOOD CHOICES

DAY 4

Breakfast: _____

Lunch: _____

Dinner: _____

Snacks: _____

PHYSICAL ACTIVITY   steps/miles/minutes: _____ | **SPIRITUAL ACTIVITY**

description: _____ | description: _____

FOOD CHOICES

DAY 5

Breakfast: _____

Lunch: _____

Dinner: _____

Snacks: _____

PHYSICAL ACTIVITY   steps/miles/minutes: _____ | **SPIRITUAL ACTIVITY**

description: _____ | description: _____

FOOD CHOICES

DAY 6

Breakfast: _____

Lunch: _____

Dinner: _____

Snacks: _____

PHYSICAL ACTIVITY   steps/miles/minutes: _____ | **SPIRITUAL ACTIVITY**

description: _____ | description: _____

FOOD CHOICES

DAY 7

Breakfast: _____

Lunch: _____

Dinner: _____

Snacks: _____

PHYSICAL ACTIVITY   steps/miles/minutes: _____ | **SPIRITUAL ACTIVITY**

description: _____ | description: _____

100-MILE CLUB

WALKING			
slowly, 2 mph	30 min =	156 cal =	1 mile
moderately, 3 mph	20 min =	156 cal =	1 mile
very briskly, 4 mph	15 min =	156 cal =	1 mile
speed walking	10 min =	156 cal =	1 mile
up stairs	13 min =	159 cal =	1 mile
RUNNING / JOGGING			
. . .	10 min =	156 cal =	1 mile
CYCLE OUTDOORS			
slowly, < 10 mph	20 min =	156 cal =	1 mile
light effort, 10-12 mph	12 min =	156 cal =	1 mile
moderate effort, 12-14 mph	10 min =	156 cal =	1 mile
vigorous effort, 14-16 mph	7.5 min =	156 cal =	1 mile
very fast, 16-19 mph	6.5 min =	152 cal =	1 mile
SPORTS ACTIVITIES			
playing tennis (singles)	10 min =	156 cal =	1 mile
swimming			
light to moderate effort	11 min =	152 cal =	1 mile
fast, vigorous effort	7.5 min =	156 cal =	1 mile
softball	15 min =	156 cal =	1 mile
golf	20 min =	156 cal =	1 mile
rollerblading	6.5 min =	152 cal =	1 mile
ice skating	11 min =	152 cal =	1 mile
jumping rope	7.5 min =	156 cal =	1 mile
basketball	12 min =	156 cal =	1 mile
soccer (casual)	15 min =	159 min =	1 mile
AROUND THE HOUSE			
mowing grass	22 min =	156 cal =	1 mile
mopping, sweeping, vacuuming	19.5 min =	155 cal =	1 mile
cooking	40 min =	160 cal =	1 mile
gardening	19 min =	156 cal =	1 mile
housework (general)	35 min =	156 cal =	1 mile

AROUND THE HOUSE			
ironing	45 min =	153 cal =	1 mile
raking leaves	25 min =	150 cal =	1 mile
washing car	23 min =	156 cal =	1 mile
washing dishes	45 min =	153 cal =	1 mile
AT THE GYM			
stair machine	8.5 min =	155 cal =	1 mile
stationary bike			
slowly, 10 mph	30 min =	156 cal =	1 mile
moderately, 10-13 mph	15 min =	156 cal =	1 mile
vigorously, 13-16 mph	7.5 min =	156 cal =	1 mile
briskly, 16-19 mph	6.5 min =	156 cal =	1 mile
elliptical trainer	12 min =	156 cal =	1 mile
weight machines (vigorously)	13 min =	152 cal =	1 mile
aerobics			
low impact	15 min =	156 cal =	1 mile
high impact	12 min =	156 cal =	1 mile
water	20 min =	156 cal =	1 mile
pilates	15 min =	156 cal =	1 mile
raquetball (casual)	15 min =	156 cal =	1 mile
stretching exercises	25 min =	150 cal =	1 mile
weight lifting (also works for weight machines used moderately or gently)	30 min =	156 cal =	1 mile
FAMILY LEISURE			
playing piano	37 min =	155 cal =	1 mile
jumping rope	10 min =	152 cal =	1 mile
skating (moderate)	20 min =	152 cal =	1 mile
swimming			
moderate	17 min =	156 cal =	1 mile
vigorous	10 min =	148 cal =	1 mile
table tennis	25 min =	150 cal =	1 mile
walk / run / play with kids	25 min =	150 cal =	1 mile

Let's Count Our Miles!

Color each circle to represent a mile you've completed.
Watch your progress to that 100 mile marker!

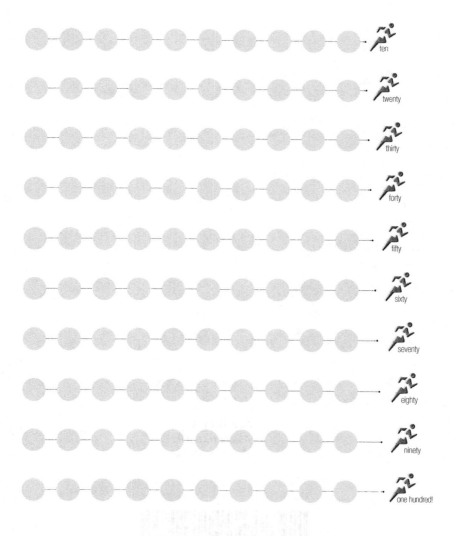

Made in the USA
Middletown, DE
22 August 2024

58983216R00126